The Big Book of Sex Toys

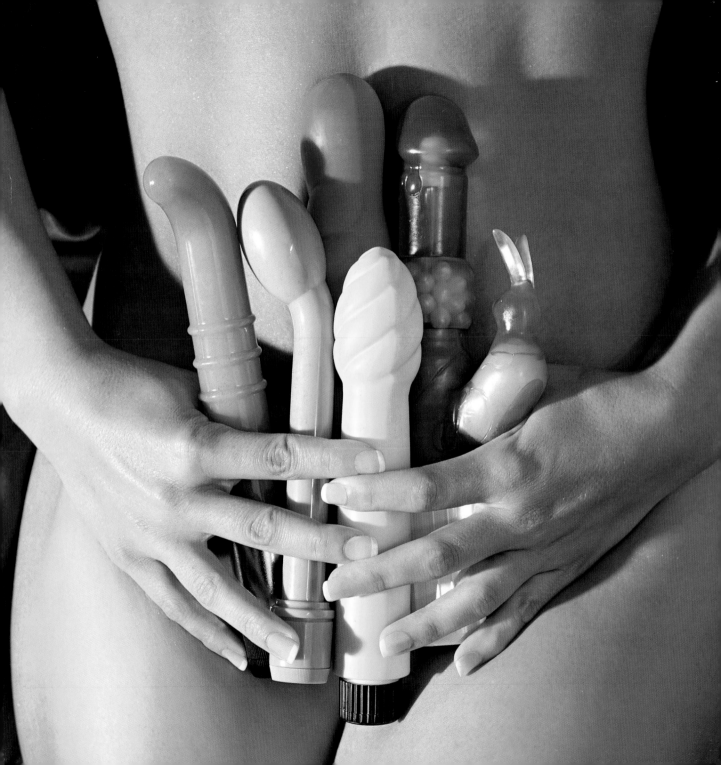

THE
BIG
BOOK
OF SEX
TOYS

From Vibrators and Dildos to Swings
and Slings—Playful and Kinky Bedside
Accessories That Make Your Sex Life Amazing

Tristan Taormino

QUIVER

Text © 2009 Tristan Taormino
Photography © 2009 Quiver

First published in the USA in 2009 by
Quiver, a member of
Quayside Publishing Group
100 Cummings Center
Suite 406-L
Beverly, MA 01915-6101
www.quiverbooks.com

The Publisher maintains the records relating to images in this book required
by 18 USC 2257. Records are located at Rockport Publishers, Inc.,
100 Cummings Center, Suite 406-L, Beverly, MA 01915-6101.

13 12 11 10 09 1 2 3 4 5

ISBN-13: 978-1-59233-355-4
ISBN-10: 1-59233-355-9

Library of Congress Cataloging-in-Publication Data

Taormino, Tristan, 1971-

The big book of sex toys : from vibrators and dildos to swings and slings-playful and
kinky bedside accessories that make your sex life amazing / [Tristan Taormino].

   p. cm.

ISBN-13: 978-1-59233-355-4
ISBN-10: 1-59233-355-9

1. Sex toys. 2. Sex instruction. 3. Sexual excitement. I. Title.

HQ31.T27195 2009

613.9'6--dc22

                                      2009021135

Cover and book design: Traffic
Book layout: Rachel Fitzgibbon
All photos courtesy of Lucia Scarlotta, except images on pages 195, courtesy of
Sportsheets International; 218–221 courtesy of Liberator Shapes; 222 and 223
courtesy of Stockroom.com.

Printed and bound in Singapore

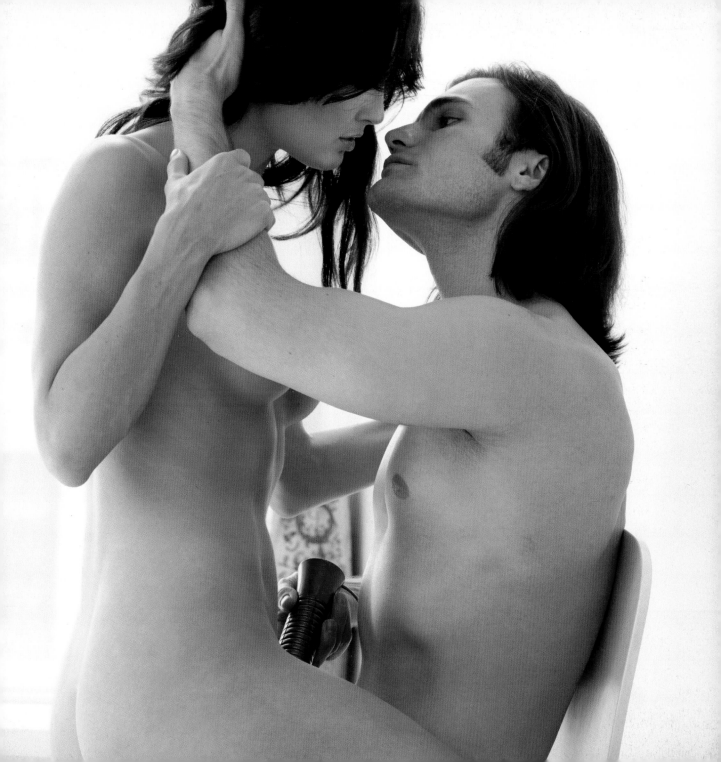

CONTENTS

OUT OF THE SHADOWS:

Sex Toys Move in to the Mainstream

Picture this: You're strolling the aisles of a well-lit, gorgeously designed boutique, which has been carefully stocked with a wide range of products—everything from classic pieces to modern high-tech trends. To your left is a long row of boxes of a product you've always wondered about but never knew whom to ask.

One has been unwrapped, is plugged in, and sits on the shelf, ready for the inquisitive consumer to pick it up, examine it, and even turn it on. You stand and read the packaging, then take a closer look at the real thing. If you have questions, the owner of the boutique, a friendly woman who greeted you when you entered, is ready to offer helpful shopping tips (from experience—she's tried most of the products herself).

So, where are you? If you haven't been into one in recent years you might be surprised to hear that what I'm describing is actually a sex toy store. In years past, adult toy stores had a much seedier image of rundown buildings in sketchy neighborhoods, windows blacked out, and neon signs screaming "XXX." The inside view wasn't much better. There, you'd most likely find racks of shrink-wrapped pink dongs labeled with words like SHAFT and INTRUDER, boxes with glossy photographs of girls whose open mouths gave no hint of what might be inside, and other items hung out of reach or tucked inside a glass counter in front of a guy you didn't want to look at, let alone ask for help. Not surprisingly, that atmosphere of sleaze and shame repelled a lot of people, especially women, whether they were shopping alone or with a partner.

Thankfully, all of that has changed dramatically. Today, whether you're curious about massage oil and feathers or dildos and bondage, you can find a clean, well-lit store where you're greeted by friendly, knowledgeable salespeople who will answer questions, give recommendations, and encourage you to stay a while and look around. Harsh fluorescent bulbs and bachelor party gag gifts have been replaced by tasteful track lighting and well-made, staff-tested toys and accessories in a couples-friendly atmosphere. Toys are out in the open for you to look at, touch, and turn on, so you can see how loud that vibrator sounds, how well made that glass dildo is, how heavy the stainless steel butt plug feels.

Nowadays, you can find couples-friendly and sex-positive stores around the country, in small and large cities as well as the suburbs. Not only do they sell erotic wares, but they also educate customers, create a safe space for people to explore their sexuality without shame, and promote a positive attitude about sex. You can also socialize with your friends at a house party and sip cocktails while you sample the latest flavored lube and examine the newest rabbit vibrator. And, for those folks not ready to venture into public or semipublic spaces, online sex shops provide people the opportunity to shop for intimate items with discretion and anonymity.

Such sex-positive sex toy shopping has changed the way we think about not only sex toys but also our own sexuality. These changes have contributed to a growing sex toy industry that is estimated to generate more than $1 billion a year—and shows no signs of slowing down. And best of all, the selection of toys available to us is bigger, more diverse, and of higher quality than ever before. While adult novelty giants like Doc Johnson and California Exotics still continue to churn out a huge selection of mass-produced toys each year, small boutique companies such as Jimmyjane and Njoy focus on a smaller number of high-end luxury toys. As a result of unique companies like theirs, many sex toys are now made with higher quality materials in aesthetically pleasing and highly functional designs.

Given all this, you might assume that the stereotypes and myths associated with sex toys would be a thing of the past. Not so! Sadly, myths still abound and prevent some people from considering what a wonderful addition toys can be to their sex lives.

Debunking Myths about Toys

1. Toys are for people who can't get "the real thing."

This myth evokes the stereotypical sex toy: the blow-up doll. It's based on the notion that the only people who buy sex toys are those who don't have a sexual partner or—worse yet—can't get one (think antisocial loners and weirdos). Their only option for sexual pleasure is to use a toy as a "replacement" for a human being. Sex toys are not replacements for partners, and people don't always use them instead of having sex. People from all walks of life, both single and partnered, use sex toys.

2. Toys are only for masturbation.

This myth is related to the first one and reinforces the idea that you only use toys by yourself. Sex toys are wonderful for solo pleasure, but they aren't just for that special alone time! There are so many different kinds of toys, and most of them can be used not only alone, but also to bring fun, fantasy, variety, and inspiration to sex with your partner.

3. Toys are for folks who have sexual problems.

This myth originated in the days when doctors diagnosed women with sexual frigidity (and other nonsexual ailments) and prescribed vibrators to induce orgasms. It was helped along by the concept of "marital aids"—the old term used to describe sex toys—a phrase that persists to this day. The underlying theme here is that toys are made to fix problems and if you're healthy, you don't need them. What a load of bull! Although toys can certainly help people with a variety of sexual issues, from low libido to erectile dysfunction, that's not their only purpose.

4. If my wife gets her hands on a vibrator, she won't need me anymore.

They may not admit it out loud, but somewhere in the back of their minds, many men have this irrational fear: a vibrator does a better job than they do. Because of this, for some, vibrators and other sex toys feel threatening. But they shouldn't. Sex toys don't put a dent in your masculinity or one-up your lovemaking skills. This is not an either/or choice or a contest. Besides, a vibrator doesn't keep her warm at night, take her to dinner, or fix things around the house!

5. If we have to use a toy, then something's wrong.

If a person feels threatened by sex toys, he may believe that his partner's desire for a toy is a not-so-subtle comment on his skill as a lover. When I worked at a sex toy store, I often met customers who resisted buying a toy by saying, "I can satisfy my partner just fine on my own—I don't need any help." Using a toy is not about compensating for your short-comings (or someone else's); it's about bringing something new into the mix to enhance sex.

For people who have gotten past the myths—and recognize that sex toys can be an incredible way to explore new dimensions of partnered and solo sex—there's just one not-so-small problem: How and what do you choose?

I wrote this book as a way to introduce people to all the different types of sex toys, and their style, form, and function. Not only is it a guidebook, but it also offers my recommendations for top toys in each category. Plus, there's advice about how to use different toys, accessories, and products to inspire, expand, and enhance your sex life. I've also included general prices, although do keep in mind that price may vary depending on where you buy.

Just as technology has revolutionized our everyday lives, I believe sex toys have the potential to transform our sex lives. I hope this book inspires you to join the revolution!

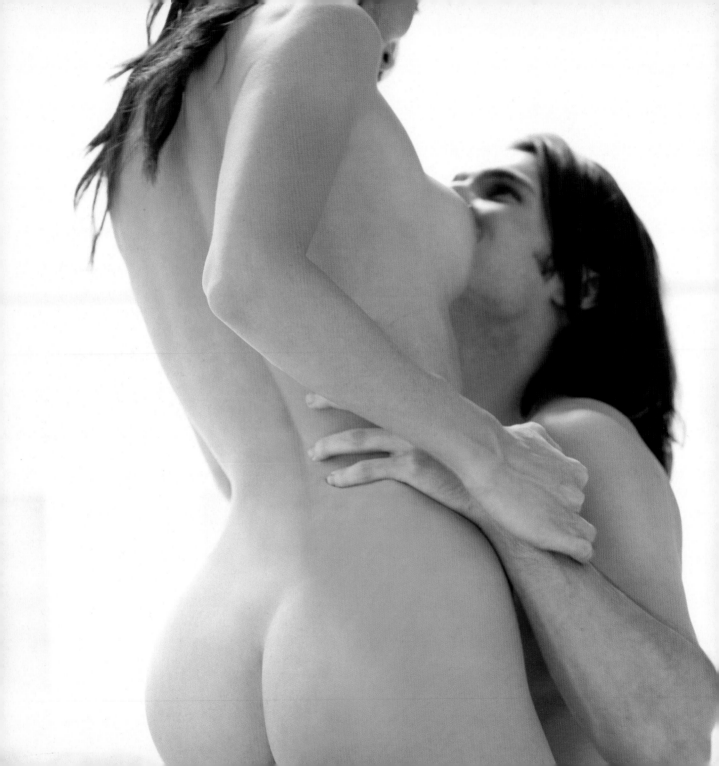

CHAPTER 1

SEXUAL ANATOMY:

Your Key To Pertinent Parts

Before we dive into the toy box, let's have a refresher course on male and female sexual anatomy. Although this chapter focuses on the genitals, know that our bodies are full of erogenous zones, and which spots are hot differ from person to person. Men and women's nipples, breasts, and chests are incredibly sensitive, and many people love to have them stimulated during sex. A well-placed stroke against the inner thighs or back of the knees, a nibble on an ear, kisses on the neck, and even stimulation of the feet can all be a big turn-on for people. So, while many of the toys in this book were designed for the vulva, anus, and penis—and those are the parts we'll cover in this chapter—don't forget the rest. Think of the entire body as your erotic canvas and sex toys as tools to help bring a sexual masterpiece to life.

Female Sexual Anatomy

The vulva encompasses the outer labia, inner labia, fourchette, frenulum, urethral opening, vaginal opening, clitoral hood, and clitoral glans. Some people refer to the vagina to describe the entire external genital region, but that's not correct. *Vulva* is the proper term, and one I use throughout the book. The outer labia (also known as the labia majora) are the outer lips of the vulva. They contain hair follicles and are naturally hairy. The outer labia are sensitive, and you can stroke, rub, lick, and even tug gently on them. The inner labia (also known as the labia minora) are the two hairless inner lips of the vulva. They can be thin and narrow, thick and wide, one of each, or somewhere in between. The inner labia tend to be more sensitive than the outer labia. When a woman is turned on, they swell and deepen in color. It's important to know that every woman's vulva is different: Some have large outer lips and thin inner ones, and some have inner lips that are much more pronounced than their outer lips. Some women's lips are similar in size, and some are asymmetrical. The skin where the inner lips meet at the bottom is a delicate spot called the fourchette. The skin where the inner lips meet at the top is the frenulum, and this can be a very sensitive spot for many women, especially because of its proximity to the clitoral glans and hood.

The clitoral hood is the skin that protects the clitoral glans; it's similar to the foreskin on a man's penis. Under the hood is the clitoral glans. The clitoral glans—which some people refer to simply as the clitoris—is the most sensitive part of a woman's body. It contains 6,000 to 8,000 nerve endings. It's important to note that the clitoris is not just this tiny nub, but also a complex system of connected nerves, tissues, muscles, and ligaments. Beneath the hood, the clitoris has a shaft, which runs from the glans to the bottom of the frenulum. The legs of the clitoris are like two ends of a wishbone and span from the shaft all the way to the fourchette.

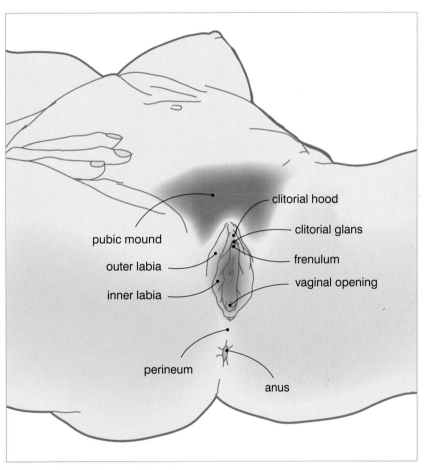

Female sexual anatomy

Below the clitoral glans and between the inner labia is the urethral opening. Behind the pubic bone is the urethra, which is about 1½ to 2 inches (3.75 to 5 cm) long and leads to the bladder. Below the urethral opening is the opening of the vagina, which is the most sensitive part of the vagina and leads to the vaginal canal.

Just inside the vaginal opening about 1 to 2 inches, through the front vaginal wall, you can feel the urethral sponge, commonly called the G-spot. The urethral sponge is made of spongy erectile tissue, which contains paraurethral glands and ducts. Like the clitoris, the G-spot is not just an isolated spot of sensitivity, but part of a network of nerves, muscles, and tissue. When a woman is turned on, the glands within the urethral sponge fill with fluid, causing the sponge to swell. Sometimes, that fluid is released through the paraurethral ducts into the urethra (or two ducts that are just adjacent to the urethra). This is called female or vaginal ejaculation.

The area between the vagina and the anus is the perineum, a sensitive but sometimes overlooked erogenous zone on the body that responds well to massage and stimulation.

Male Sexual Anatomy

The scrotal sac is the sac of skin that surrounds the testicles. The testicles, commonly called the balls, are the glands involved in the production of testosterone and sperm. The shaft is the main body of the penis. The glans, also called the head, is the most sensitive part of a man's penis because it has the most nerve endings. The urethral opening is the hole where urine and ejaculate leave the body.

On a circumcised penis, the foreskin has been removed so that the head is always visible. The corona—sometimes referred to as the coronal ridge—is the outer perimeter of the head that joins the

head to the shaft. If you follow the ridge of the corona to the underside of the penis, you'll notice where the two ends come together: This is the frenulum. This area is often the most sensitive part of the head.

An uncircumcised penis has a foreskin, a sheath of skin that covers and protects the glans. The foreskin's inside fold is made of mucous membrane and keeps the surface of the glans soft, moist, and sensitive. The foreskin contains a rich supply of blood vessels and a dense concentration of nerve endings. The frenulum on an uncircumcised penis is where the foreskin attaches to the head on the underside.

The perineum is the area between the base of the penis and the anal opening. When you stimulate a man's perineum, you're stimulating the bulb of the penis, the part that extends inside his body.

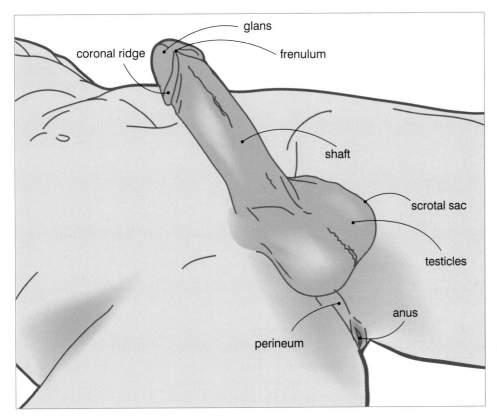

Male sexual anatomy

Anal Anatomy

Men and women have nearly identical anorectal anatomy, so the following applies to you regardless of your gender. The anus is the anal opening; it is made of soft tissue that is rich in nerve endings. It has a puckered appearance, and the skin around it contains hair follicles.

Just inside the anus are the external and internal sphincter muscles. These are the muscles that give the anus that tight feeling and control bowel movements; they are the ones we must learn to relax in order to achieve comfortable anal penetration. Closer to the opening is the external sphincter. You can learn to control the external sphincter, making it tense or relax. Imagine that you are holding something in your ass or expelling something. As you suck in and tense up or push down and release, you are exercising your external sphincter muscles. The internal sphincter, on the other hand, is controlled by the autonomic nervous system, which also controls such involuntary bodily functions as your breathing rate. This muscle ordinarily reacts reflexively; for example,

when you are ready to have a bowel movement, the internal sphincter relaxes, allowing feces to move from the rectum to the anal canal and out the anus. The external and the internal sphincter muscles can work independently of each other, but because they overlap, they often work together. The more aware you are of your sphincters and the more you practice using them, the more toned and "in shape" they will be, and the easier and more comfortable anal penetration will be.

The anal canal is the first few inches inside the anus, and is made of soft, sensitive tissue with a high concentration of nerve endings. Beyond the anal canal is the rectum, which is 8 to 9 inches (20 to 22.5 cm) long; the rectum is made up of loose folds of soft, smooth tissue. Wider than the anal canal, the rectum has the ability to expand more than the anal canal when you are aroused, which is what makes penetration possible.

The rectum is not a straight tube, but has two gentle curves. The lower part of the rectum curves toward your navel. After a few inches, the rectum curves back

toward your spine, then toward your navel again. The rectum and colon both curve laterally (from side to side) as well; whether they curve to the right or the left will vary from person to person. These curves are part of the reason that anal penetration should be slow and gentle, especially at first. Each person's rectum and its curves are unique, and it is best to feel your way inside the rectum slowly, following its curves, rather than jamming anything straight inside.

The anus, the anal canal, and the rectum are all sensitive in different ways, which is why anal stimulation and penetration can be so pleasurable. The anus and the outer part of the anal canal are made of the same sensitive soft tissue, and this tissue contains the highest concentration of nerve endings of all our anal anatomy. In general, this tissue tends to be more sensitive to touch and vibration. The inner part of the anal canal and the rectum are made of mucous membrane and have a lot fewer nerve endings; however, this tissue is much more sensitive to pressure (from penetration, for example).

When it comes to anorectal anatomy, the one important difference between men and women is that men have a prostate gland. The prostate gland (sometimes referred to as the P-spot or the male G-spot) surrounds part of a man's urethra; it's behind the pubic bone, below the bladder and above the base of the penis. A mass of muscle, glands, and connective tissue, the prostate is about the size and shape of a walnut; it produces ejaculatory fluid that combines with sperm and fluid from the seminal vesicles to create male ejaculate. The prostate gland is 1 to 2 inches (2.5 to 5 cm) inside a man's anus on the front wall, so it can be directly stimulated through anal penetration. Prostate stimulation can be incredibly pleasurable, and many men can have an orgasm from prostate stimulation alone or combined with genital stimulation. Women lack a prostate gland, but many still find anal sex pleasurable.

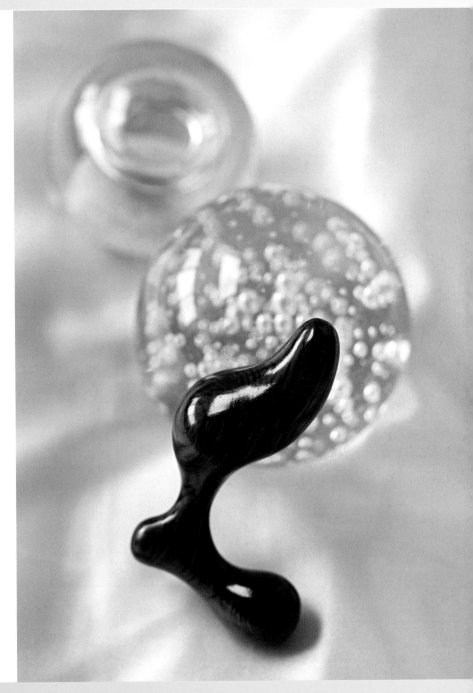

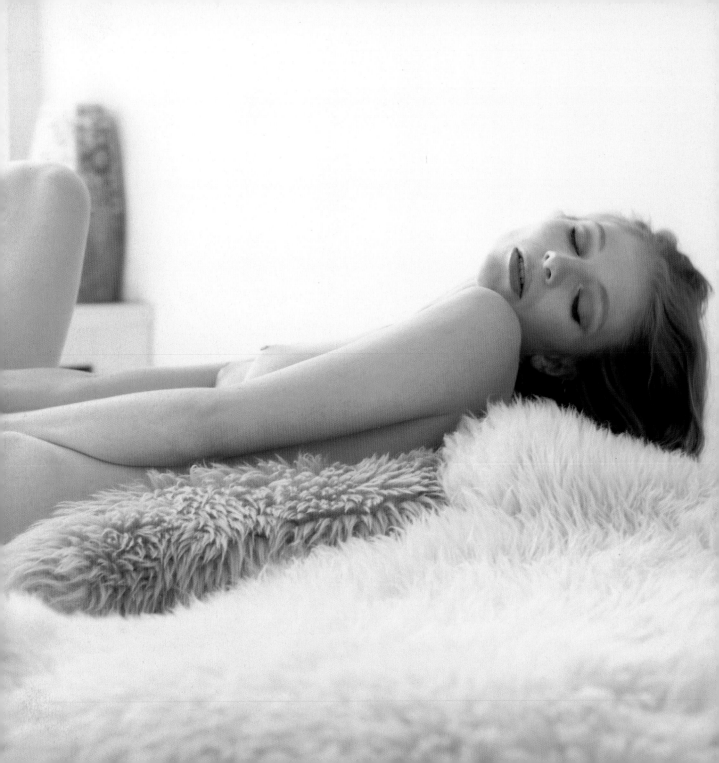

CHAPTER 2

SEX TOYS: Your Path to Solo *and* Partnered Pleasure

For many people, the first sexual partner we have is ourselves, and masturbation is the way we get to know our sexual selves. As we touch ourselves, we explore our bodies, discover new sensations, and try different techniques. Masturbation is a gift, an act of self-love. People masturbate with different intentions and for different reasons: to have an orgasm, to fantasize, to melt away stress, to help fall asleep (or wake up), or to feel a connection to your own body. Using a toy while you masturbate is a good way to learn about your body and your sexuality, strengthen and tone your pelvic muscles, spice up your routine, and explore a new activity.

Solo Play: Self-Discovery Equals Better Sex

Most boys begin to masturbate when they hit puberty; their first erection, wet dream, and masturbation session are all rites of passage in our society. By the time they are young adults, they've explored how their penis works and have masturbated to orgasm. On the other hand, many girls don't have a parallel experience. A girl's first clitoral hard-on isn't exactly a common theme in pop culture. And women aren't encouraged to embrace their sexual bodies in the same way that men are. As a result, many women don't masturbate regularly or have never masturbated at all. This double standard puts women at a great disadvantage in their sexual evolution, and they often grow up with feelings of ambivalence, guilt, confusion, or shame about their own bodies.

For a woman who's never masturbated before, a sex toy like a vibrator is a great way to introduce her to the idea. If she feels shy about touching herself or insecure about what to do, a vibrator can lend the helping, um, hand she needs. Similarly, for women who've never had an orgasm or who have trouble reaching orgasm, a vibrator is often recommended by sex therapists and physicians.

Regardless of your gender, self-discovery shouldn't end once you become sexually active. When people ask me for tips on how to become a better lover, I have one piece of advice for everyone: masturbate. That's right: The more you have sex with yourself, the better you'll be at having sex with your partner. Self-knowledge is the key to sexual health, well-being, and pleasure. And the more you know about your own body—what you like, what you don't, what feels good, what doesn't, what turns you on, what turns you off—the more you can share with your partner.

Using a toy while you masturbate is also a good way to try out something new. Perhaps you're interested in experiment-ing—with using a vibrator, testing out a cock ring, or exploring anal penetration. Whatever it is, it may be something you're curious about, but you're not ready to discuss it or try it out with your partner. *That's okay.*You don't have to share every sexual desire you have with your partner right away. Instead, give it a try during a solo session, and see how you like it. Perhaps you'll decide to keep it to yourself, reserving it for self-pleasuring occasions. Or you may find that you like it so much that you want to share it with your partner.

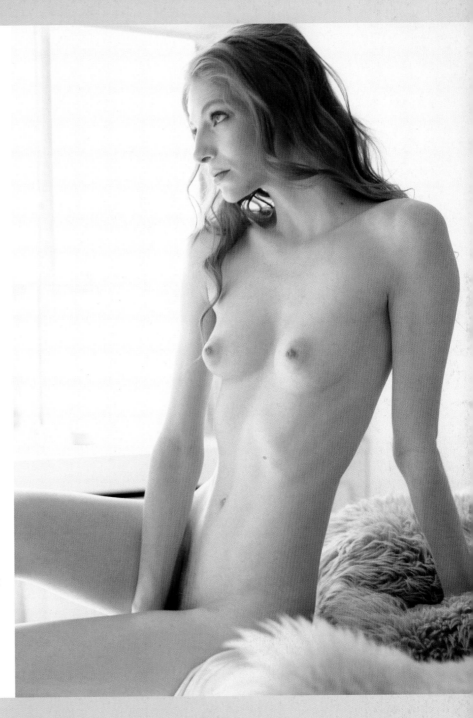

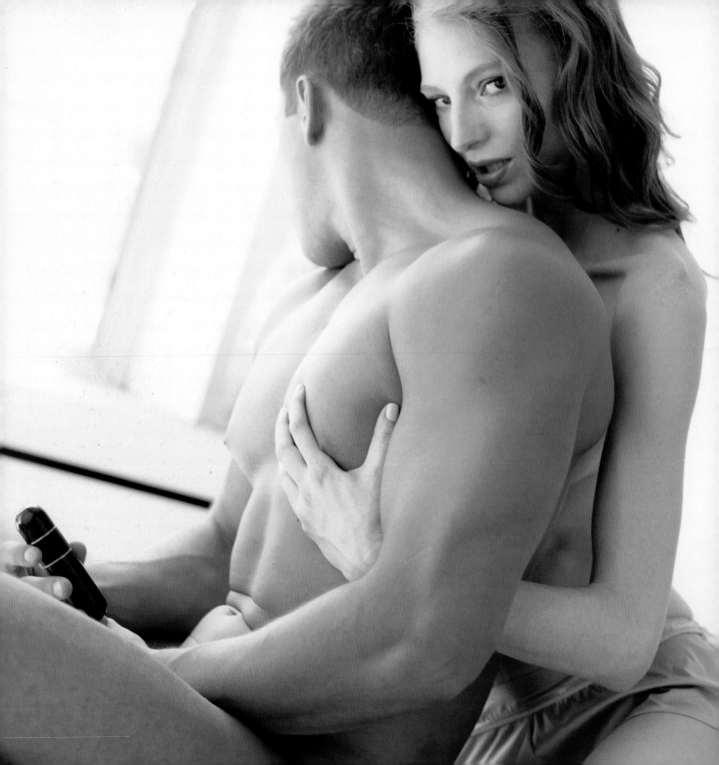

Sexual Exercise for Better Health

Masturbation isn't just fun, it's actually good for you! Just as we know that exercise is good for our bodies and helps reduce the risk of certain conditions and illnesses, exercising our sexual anatomy is also important. Specifically, exercising the pubococcygeus muscles (also known as the PC muscles) plays a big role in men and women's sexual health. The PC muscles run from the pubic bone to the tailbone, supporting the uterus, bladder, and bowel. For men and women alike, these muscles contract randomly when you are sexually aroused and rhythmically during orgasm. By toning and strengthening the PC muscles through exercise, men can improve prostate health, learn to control and delay ejaculation, control incontinence, maintain better erections, and experience more sensitivity during sex.

For women, the PC muscles can be stressed, weakened, or atrophied from obesity, during pregnancy and childbirth, after a period of sexual abstinence, or just as part of the aging process. By exercising and strengthening your PC muscles, you can get better in tune with the feelings in your pelvic area, increasing your sensitivity and responsiveness. The exercises will also tone the pelvic muscles, making them more flexible and more receptive to pleasurable sensations. Women who regularly exercise their PC and pelvic muscles report it helps them:

- Maintain urinary tract health

- Prevent or control incontinence

- Prepare for pregnancy and childbirth

- Achieve greater sensitivity during sex

- Have increased pleasure during clitoral stimulation and vaginal and anal penetration

- Have better, more controlled orgasms

Kegel exercises were named for the physician who first popularized the theory of exercising PC muscles. You can do the exercises lying down, sitting, or standing, and doing them during masturbation will increase blood flow to the genitals and increase your arousal. As with other exercise regimens, this should be performed daily for best results. If your muscles seem tired at first, don't worry—that's normal. The harder the exercises are to do for you, the less toned your PC muscles are, and the more you need a workout. Use your common sense, and don't overdo it to begin with; if you experience any pain while doing them, see a doctor.

To locate your PC muscles, imagine that you are trying to stop peeing (or while you are peeing, you can actually stop the flow of urine). The muscles you contract to stop the flow are your PC muscles. You can also slide a finger inside your vagina and try to squeeze your finger with your muscles. Once you've found the PC muscles, take some deep breaths. Contract the muscles and hold the contraction for a few seconds. Then relax the muscles. Begin to add a second to the routine, and see whether you can work your way up to 10 seconds of contraction followed by 10 seconds of relaxation. You can do these in sets of ten several times a day. For best results, make sure you're isolating the PC muscle. Don't hold your breath or contract your stomach or other muscles.

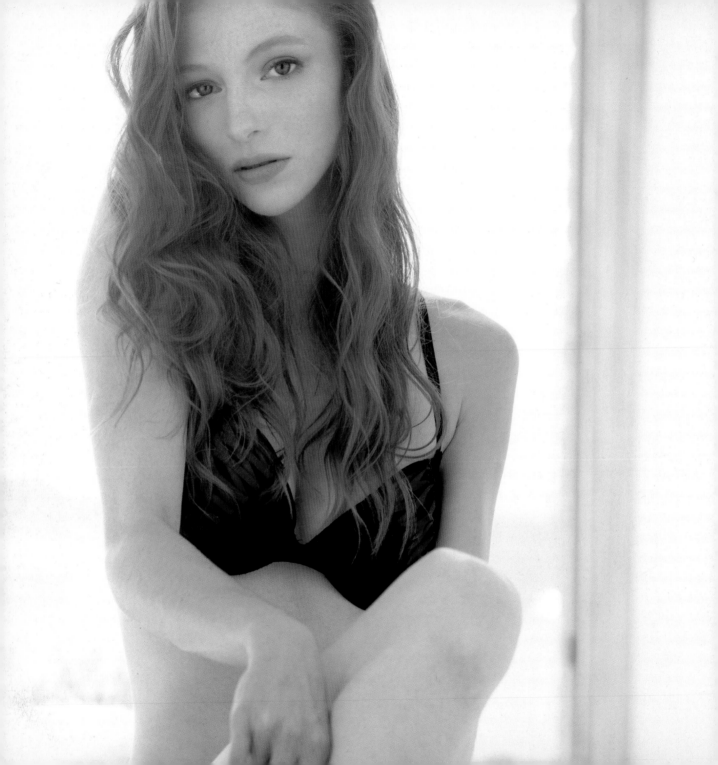

Vaginal Exercise: Try Ben-Wa Balls, Stone Eggs, and Barbells

Some people believe that doing PC muscle exercises with something inside the vagina (or in the anus for men) produces better results because you're working the muscles against some resistance. There are several products designed especially for Kegel exercises.

Large egg-shaped toys made of polished jade, onyx, and other natural stones can be used by women to exercise your PC muscles. You slide a well-lubed egg into your vagina, then practice contracting your muscles around it. Because it's both thick and heavy, it provides more of a challenge to the muscles. Once the muscles are stronger, you can do the exercises standing up. Smaller and lighter than stone eggs, Ben-Wa balls are two balls on a string usually made of plastic or silicone. They are a good starter for people intimidated by the size and weight of the egg. Eggs and Ben-Wa balls should not be used anally.

Heavier but not as thick as eggs, vaginal barbells are recommended by physicians, sexologists, and therapists for Kegel exercises. The Kegelcisor and Betty's Vaginal Barbell (designed by masturbation guru and sexologist Betty Dodson) are heavy metal dildos that are similar in design: They are about 7 inches (18 cm) long, weigh nearly a pound, and have different-sized balls on either end. You begin by practicing clamping down on the larger ball, then graduate to the smaller one as your muscle tone improves; some exercises call for you to contract the muscle while pulling the barbell out of your vagina. The Natural Contours Energie is a similar product, except it has a plastic coating over metal and a smooth surface without balls. All three can be used anally, but with great caution, because they don't have flared bases. When the workout is over, the barbells, Ben-Wa balls, and stone egg can also be used as sex toys, just for pleasure.

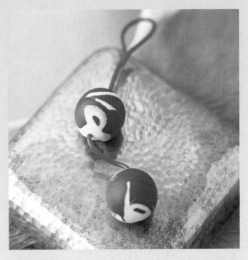

Ben-Wa Balls

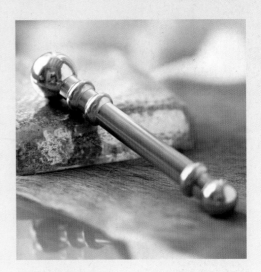

Betty's Vaginal Barbell

Partnered Pleasure Gets an Assist

Sex toys are designed for pleasure, and your sex life can benefit from them in many different ways. Although toys have come a long way since they were considered "marital aids," one thing remains true: They *can* be problem solvers. Low libido is one of the most common issues that women face, especially as they get older. For women who have trouble getting aroused, a vibrator can help get the party started. For men, erectile dysfunction and premature ejaculation are two of the most common problems. Penis pumps can help you get an erection; a cock ring can help you maintain a stronger erection, delay ejaculation, and prolong intercourse.

One of the most common complaints I hear from women is that there isn't enough foreplay before intercourse. In general, it takes women more time than men to get aroused. If you have inter-course before you're properly warmed up, your body literally isn't ready: The genitals aren't fully engorged, and the vagina hasn't lubricated and expanded. Some women who experience pain during intercourse simply haven't given their bodies enough time to rev up. All sorts of sex toys, including dildos and vibrators, can be used to facilitate the arousal process. They can help make foreplay fun and playful, relax you, and get you in the mood. In addition, if your partner is well endowed, penetration with a toy that's slightly smaller than him is a great way to prepare.

Sex toys can also give you an "extra set of hands" in the bedroom, allowing you to do two or three things (or be in two or three places) at once! Imagine if you could give her vaginal penetration, clitoral stimulation, and anal pleasure simultane-ously. You can with a butt plug, a vibrator, or a dildo to help you out. When the perfect position for intercourse means you can't reach other parts of her body, a vibrator can be there for you. What if you want to play with his penis, balls, and nipples at the same time? Nipple clamps and a small vibrator will help you cover all his hot spots.

I like to think of sex toys as tools for evolution: They expand your sexual repertoire. One of the best things about sex toys is that they can help you move away from an intercourse-always model of sex. Intercourse is often seen as the ultimate activity, the one you're working your way toward, the main event. But the truth is that intercourse isn't the only way to have sex. Some folks prefer other kinds of pleasure, including mutual masturbation, manual stimulation, and oral sex. Some women can't orgasm from intercourse. Some people can't have intercourse. Women with high-risk pregnancies, those who've just given birth, and those with certain medical conditions may not be able to have intercourse, just as men with erectile dysfunction or prostate issues may not.

But that doesn't mean you can't have sex! Toys give couples the opportunity to think outside the box.

Research has shown that the majority of women need clitoral stimulation to orgasm. For some women, a hand or a tongue simply is not enough. They need a powerful, focused, consistent kind of stimulation that human beings can't always provide. That's why vibrators exist! Vibrators deliver a particular type of stimulation that is unmatched. Some women find that oral sex and manual stimulation feel wonderful, turn them on, and get them to the edge, but can't deliver them into ecstasy. Vibrators can get you to the finish line.

For long-term couples, toys can be that spark you need to reignite your sexual relationship. Sometimes, when you bring something new and fresh to your sex life, it helps you reconnect with your partner. Simply shopping for a new play object can be a huge turn-on for many couples.

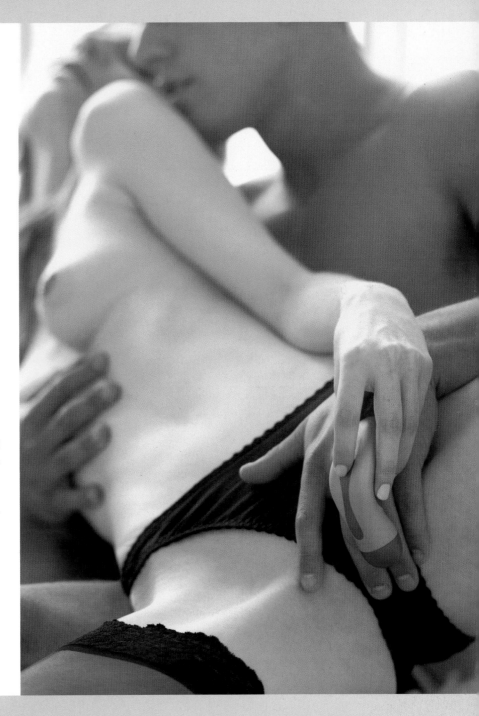

As you browse the shelves at a store, you can whisper sexy things to one another, reveal what you like about a certain toy, and tease each other with the possibilities. Once you've made your purchase, there's plenty more fun to come. Each Christmas, a man I know orders a special new toy for his wife and includes a handwritten card with it; it has become a tradition for them. He loves to figure out the perfect one to buy, while she revels in the anticipation of what's waiting for her under the tree. They've had an exciting, fulfilling sex life for more than fifteen years together.

Liberator Shapes, swings, and slings can help change the angle of penetration or support and arrange your bodies in ways you never thought possible, thus inspiring new positions. Items such as blindfolds, massage oil candles, and G-spot toys may introduce new activities into your erotic repertoire. Toys can also set the stage for fantasy role-playing; sometimes all it takes is a crack of the paddle to keep naughty girls or boys in line! Ultimately, there's a reason vibrators, dildos, and plugs are called sex *toys*: They're lots of fun!

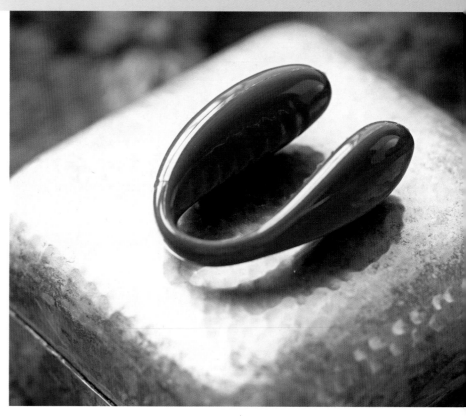

The We-Vibe (see page 88)

Top Ten Reasons to Add Sex Toys to Your Sex Life

1. Explore something new: It's easy to get bored or complacent in a long-term sexual relationship. Kick things up a notch with a sex toy.

2. Go from good to great: Already having hot sex? Put technology and innovation to work for you, and make it even hotter.

3. Have a quickie: Sometimes, you just need to get off and get off quick. Why not take a shortcut to that release and relaxation?

4. Show and tell: Take turns masturbating for each other, each with a favorite toy. You'll get to watch each other, show off for your partner, and maybe learn a thing or two about your lover from the performance.

5. Stay up all night: Let's say your penis is done for the evening, but the two of you aren't. Grab a toy, and you're good to go for as many more rounds as you want.

6. Bring her over the edge: Some women need powerful, nonstop clitoral stimulation to come, and a vibrator is the only thing that will help them get there.

7. Achieve synchronicity: Want to experience pleasure in all the right places at the same exact time? Simultaneous sensations (and orgasms) are possible!

8. Go for more: Whether you want to learn how to become multiorgasmic or it comes, well, naturally to you, toys help inspire multiple orgasms for him and her.

9. Double the pleasure: Is your partner craving twice the fun but you don't want to invite a neighbor over to help out? You can be both places at once with a dildo or vibrator.

10. Create your own adventure: If the bedroom is your stage, consider sex toys the props in your erotic drama; be creative, have fun, and embrace your playful side!

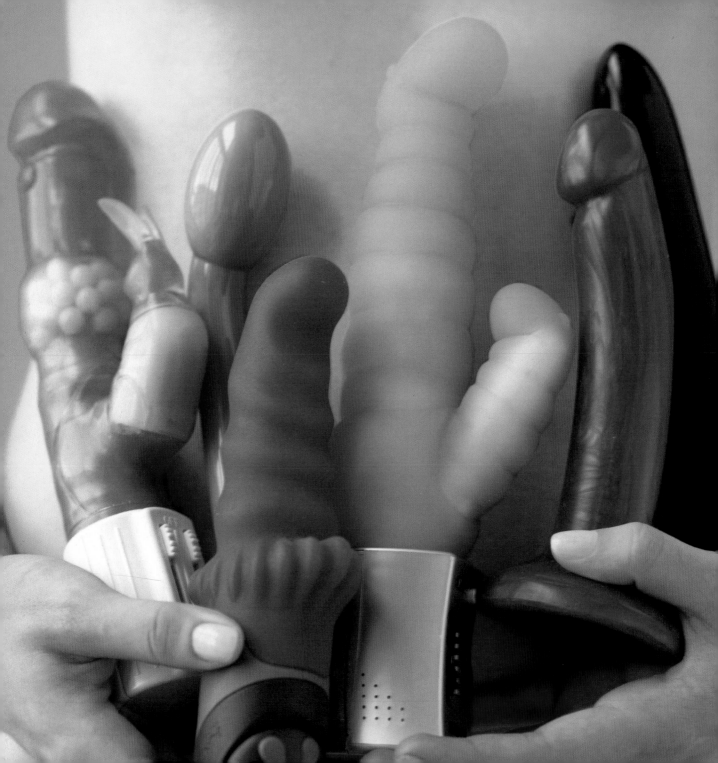

CHAPTER 3

SHOPPING:

How to Choose the Best Toys for You

There are many different factors to consider when selecting a toy, including function, style, material, size, cost, and your own personal taste. This chapter offers a good guide for what to think about before you buy; as you think about your options, keep in mind that you don't have to limit yourself to just one toy!

Consider Functionality

What would you like the toy to do? What do you want to use it for? What features are important to you? Some toys are pretty self-explanatory when it comes to figuring out what they are created for; for example, if you want to blindfold someone, you can get a blindfold. But other toys are a little more complex. Some are designed for a very specific task. An ergonomic vibrator, for instance, has a single purpose: Its shape is meant to hug the curves of a woman's body and deliver clitoral stimulation. A vaginal barbell is suitable for women who want to exercise and strengthen their PC muscles and for those who like the feeling of a heavy object inside. As its name indicates, a butt plug is an anal pleasure toy, but it delivers a specific kind of anal stimulation: a feeling of fullness inside the rectum without any movement. So, if you like in-and-out movement during anal penetration, a plug is not the best toy for the job (try a dildo instead).

Other toys can be used for several different activities, such as some vibrators. Although slimline and phallic vibrators appear to be built for penetration, they can also be used for external clitoral stimulation. Wand-style vibrators are for external stimulation only; however, many have separate attachments that transform them into insertable toys. Fingertip vibes are great for stimulating clits, and they can also bring some buzz to the nipples, anus, balls, and shaft of the penis. Curved dildos and wands are great for both G-spot and prostate stimulation. Some toys are multitaskers, such as double-ended dildos, which allow two partners to be penetrated at the same time. Similarly, dual-action vibrators are made for simultaneous vaginal penetration and clitoral stimulation. (See the sidebar for more examples.)

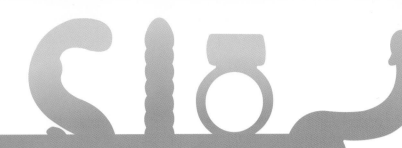

Pick Your Pleasure: Toys by Function

- External clitoral vibrators: bullets, eggs, fingertip vibes, pocket rockets, disguised vibes, ergonomic vibrators, wand-style plug-ins, wearable vibes, slimline vibes, phallic vibes, luxury vibes, smart vibes, vibrating cock rings

- Vaginal penetration with vibration: hands-free insertable vibes, slimline vibes, phallic vibes, G-spotters, luxury vibes, some smart vibes, dildos with vibrator, wand-style plug-in vibrators with attachments

- Simultaneous clitoral vibration and vaginal penetration: rabbit-style dual-action vibes, curvy double-action vibes

- Vaginal penetration (without vibration): dildos, wands, vaginal barbells

- G-spot stimulation: G-spot vibrators, luxury vibes, curved dildos, wands, wand-style plug-in vibrators with G-spot attachments

- Anal penetration with vibration: dildos with bullet vibes, vibrating butt plugs, inflatable plugs, vibrating probes

- Anal penetration: anal beads, butt plugs, dildos, curved dildos, wands

- Strap-on sex: dildos, dildos with bullet vibes, strap-on harnesses, thigh harnesses

- Simultaneous penetration for him and her: double-headed dildos, simultaneous penetration toys

- Prostate stimulation: curved dildos, some G-spot vibrators and wands, butt plugs, vibrating butt plugs, prostate toys

- Erection enhancement: cock rings, penis pumps

- Penis and ball stimulation: penis sleeves, penis pumps, vibrators, bullets, eggs, fingertip vibes, pocket rockets, wand-style plug-ins, vibrating cock rings

- Sensation play: feathers, massage oil, edible body paint and dust, massage oil candles, liquid latex

- Bondage: blindfolds, hoods, bondage tape, cuffs and restraints, collars, bondage kits

- Spanking: paddles, slappers, crops

- Role-play and fetish: nipple clamps, paddles, slappers, crops, floggers, canes

Consider Your Style

Each person has his or her own unique sense of style, and we express our taste in many different ways, from the clothes we wear, to how we style our hair, to how we decorate our homes. It used to be that the majority of sex toys were cheaply made, and they looked like garish props. Thankfully, manufacturers have come a long way in developing toys that are not only well crafted, but are also aesthetically pleasing to a variety of people with different preferences.

For some people, when it comes to their toys, it's all about realism. They want dildos and vibrators to closely resemble penises and penis sleeves to look like vaginas (and anuses). If you want a realistic-looking and -feeling toy, look for thermal plastic toys (with brand names such as CyberSkin) or silicone ones (especially the silicone material VixSkin by Vixen Creations). These materials are the closest to the feel and texture of real flesh. Realistic-style dildos and vibrators have anatomically correct circumcised heads, balls, and even veins. Many come in different skin colors. The same holds true for penis sleeves designed to look like vaginas: The more detailed (and expensive) of this variety are replicas

of female sexual anatomy, complete with inner and outer labia, clitoris, vaginal opening, and pubic hair, and some even have G-spots inside!

Other people want toys to look very discreet, the kind of object that if spotted in your luggage or on a bedside table wouldn't warrant a second glance. These often look like ordinary household gadgets, and have clean lines and simple designs. Similarly, some prefer more masculine-style toys that come in solid colors, black, or white and don't have fancy embellishments or textures. At the other end of the spectrum are folks who like playful toys: They may look like animals, vegetables, or fanciful creatures. These styles often come in bright colors, festive patterns, and charming packaging. Similarly, if you're a girly girl, there are plenty of toys out there to suit your style; think pinks, purples, reds, floral designs, leopard prints, and lots of sparkle!

One of the trends in the adult toy industry definitely reflects the technologically savvy world around us; these are toys for the iPod generation and have a decidedly modern flair. They're shiny, sleek, ergonomic, made of top-notch materials, and above all, very high-tech. Some of

them even look like toys from the future, and these are perfect for the gadget-loving super geek in your life. Another trend is the rise of boutique companies that produce a small number of very high-end luxury toys. Some are made of top-notch materials such as glass, metal, stone, ceramic, and wood, while others take it a step further to Swarovski crystals, 24-karat gold, Italian leather, jade, and pearls. Some are hand made, limited edition, or one of a kind, and their presentation and packaging is usually as decadent as the toys themselves. These toys capture a stunning design aesthetic, elevating the items from gorgeous sex toys to works of art—and they have a price tag that reflects their superior design and craftsmanship.

Other Factors to Consider: Cost, Durability, and Size

Speaking of price tags, how much are you willing to spend? Cost is definitely a factor, because toys can run anywhere from $15 (for a small vibrating egg) to hundreds of dollars for a silicone vibrator. When it comes to luxury items and sex furniture, you can even move into the thousands. Pricing is pretty consistent in the adult industry, and you generally get what you pay for. Toys made of inexpensive plastics that can be mass-produced are much less expensive than those crafted of superior materials that require more labor to create them as well as those that feature unique designs and technology. Also keep in mind that cheaper toys made of materials such as rubber/PVC should be replaced every year, whereas pricier toys should be built to last longer, depending on the material. A guide to all the different sex toy materials is in the next chapter.

When it comes to sex toys, size does matter and your individual needs will dictate what the ideal size is for you. Maybe you want a toy that you can easily fit in your purse or that won't take up too much room in your luggage. If it's a penetration toy, terms such as "small" and "large" are all relative and very individual, which is why it's a good idea to see a toy out of its packaging before you buy it (or look for measurements). Want to use your vibrator mostly by yourself, with a partner, or both? Smaller vibrators can be easier for some people to incorporate into intercourse.

Go Green: How to Shop with Mother Earth in Mind

For those of you who shudder at the thought of your old vibrators taking up space in a landfill somewhere and who want to be kinder to the Earth as you get your groove on, here are some eco-friendly sex toys and practices:

1. Buy a rechargeable vibrator over a battery-powered one.

2. Use rechargeable batteries in your battery-powered toys.

3. Look for nontoxic materials, such as medical-grade silicone, glass, metal, and phthalate-free plastics.

4. Pick materials that can be recycled, such as glass and metal.

5. Participate in a sex toy recycling program. Believe it or not, they do exist. Some stores will accept old or broken toys and give you a credit toward a new purchase.

6. Find toys made of recycled products, such as rubber whips and strap-on harnesses made from old tires.

7. Do some research to find toys that are ethically manufactured and traded.

8. Use toys made of natural materials, including sustainably harvested wood, marble, granite, and stone.

9. Choose natural and organic lubes, massage oils, and other body products, and ask whether they are tested on animals.

10. Purchase toys in eco-friendly and recyclable packaging.

Choosing a Good Sex Store by Cory Silverberg

The sad fact is that there are far more bad sex stores than good ones. A bad sex store is one that overcharges, offers little to no customer service, and sells products of questionable safety. A good sex store charges fair prices, offers basic warranties, and trains its staff so they can answer your questions honestly and intelligently (and without rolling their eyes). To some extent, finding a good sex store is about the fit, but there are some things to look for and to think about. Below are tips from one of the best people in the business: Cory Silverberg, a twenty-year veteran of sex toy retailing.

Get a recommendation. It might be embarrassing to ask a friend, but you're never going to get a more honest answer or advertisement for a sex store than the one you get from someone who has shopped there. If you don't want to ask a friend, do some online research on neighborhood review sites (such as Yelp.com).

Make them work for your business. Call a store and ask a few questions about their business or about a specific product. See how their customer service is. If they're friendly and give you their time, it's a good sign. If they're just trying to get you off the phone and seem rude, move on. I also recommend sending a store an email with a request for a product recommendation. See how long they take to respond, and whether you feel like they're pushing the most expensive products or actually listening to your question.

Know the policies. Make sure you know what their return and warranty policies are. If they don't offer at least a thirty-day warranty on defective merchandise take your business elsewhere. If they aren't clear with you about what happens if their DVD doesn't work in your player or you don't like the book you bought, think twice before giving them your business.

Compare prices. If you go online you'll find a huge range in pricing for any given product. Use the Web to do comparison shopping, but keep in mind that if you want quality customer service, and a company that will stand behind its products, you'll probably pay a little more, and it's worth it.

Shop in person. This isn't always possible, but when you shop in person you get way more information about what you're buying and whether or not it's going to be right for you. The Web is great for research, but once you know what you want, call around to see whether any sex stores in your area carry it.

Find a store that caters to your ethics. There are sex stores that focus on organic products, sex stores that are worker cooperatives, feminist sex stores, and online stores catering just to Christians. One of the great benefits of the boom in sex toy sales is that it's now easier to shop in a way that doesn't compromise your ethics and values (or at least doesn't compromise them as much!). Don't feel like you have to settle for a cheesy or sleazy porn shop, unless that's what you're looking for.

Demand real answers, not marketing. It's a good idea to ask a few questions to test the knowledge of the sales staff. Asking them to explain, for example, why one product is much more expensive than the other or what they'd recommend for a first-time vibrator should give you a sense of how much they know about their products and how they work. If the answer you get sounds more like a sales pitch than a personal and relevant response, be wary. Although more stores are training their staff, it doesn't mean they are training them well!

Follow these minimum expectations for online shopping. If you shop online, make sure the company has a toll-free number and that they will pay for shipping if you receive a defective product. If they don't have a posted policy, get something in an email from them before you shop. The same goes for a privacy policy. If it's not posted on the site, don't shop until you've got something in writing.

Cory Silverberg is a worker-owner of Come As You Are (comeasyouare.com), the world's only democratically run, worker cooperative sex toy store. He is also the Sexuality Guide for About.com (sexuality.about.com) and the coauthor of The Ultimate Guide to Sex and Disability.

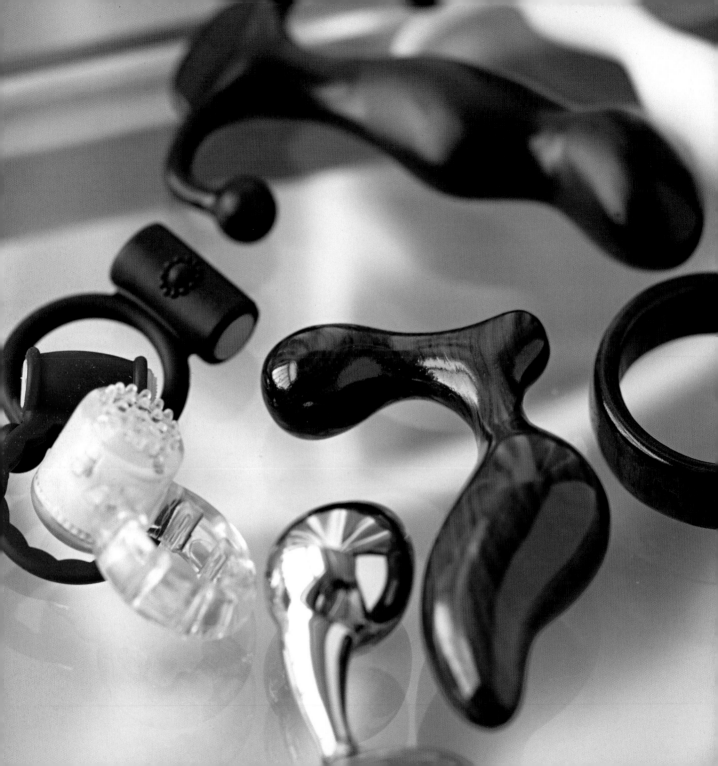

CHAPTER 4

NOT ALL SEX TOYS ARE CREATED EQUAL:

Your Primer on What They're Made Of

Many sex toys—especially inexpensive "adult novelties" found at traditional adult bookstores—are made of some kind of rubber, vinyl, or softened PVC (polyvinyl chloride, plus softening agents known as phthalates). These toys are cheap to produce and thus often very affordable.

Dildos, vibrators, butt plugs, cock rings, penis sleeves, and other toys made of these materials come in a wide variety of styles, from super-realistic flesh-toned dildos to colorful and glittery vibrators.

In recent years, there has been some serious debate about the safety of these toys, because they contain chemicals known as phthalates (see sidebar on page 44). However, companies are developing soft plastics without these chemicals, so if this is a concern for you, look for toys marked "phthalate-free." The biggest pro of soft PVC, rubber, and rubberlike materials is their price point, so if you want to try something without spending a lot of cash, this is a good bet. But these toys are not long-term investments; they definitely have a shelf life and should be replaced regularly (at least once a year). Because they are porous, you should never share these toys, or always cover them with condoms if you do.

Elastomers are flexible plastics. Some companies have turned to elastomers to make toys that look and feel like rubber but are latex-free, more resilient, and free of phthalates. Toys made of elastomers are firm yet soft, durable, and hypoallergenic. They are slightly porous, so they shouldn't be shared unless you protect them with condoms. Clean them with soap and water. Thermoplastic rubber (TPR) is also a phthalate-free soft material that has a durable yet pliable texture. It's still porous, so TPR toys should not be shared.

Thermal Plastics: Closest to Real Skin

Thermal plastic toys—sold under popular brand names such as CyberSkin, SoftSkin, Real Feel Super Skin, and UltraSkin—are soft, are very realistic looking, and come closest of all sex toy materials to feeling like skin. Although the formulas vary, thermal plastics tend to be slightly stretchy and have the same give as human flesh. Most thermal plastics do not contain phthalates, but always check the packaging or ask the retailer to make sure. There are dildos, vibrating dildos, vibrators, and penis sleeves made of thermal plastics.

The unique element of this material is that it comes very close to the feeling of skin. The drawback to these toys is that they are hard to clean and maintain. They are prone to small nicks, because the material can be quite fragile. Use only water-based lubes with these toys, because oil-based lubes will destroy them and silicone lubes can melt or degrade the material. Cleaning and caring for them properly is the key to maintaining a thermal plastic toy's pliable texture and having it last a long time.

Silicone: More Expensive, but Definitely Worth It

If you want a soft, flexible toy that's durable, easy to clean, and can be disinfected, silicone is the top-of-the-line material. That also means it's the most expensive of the soft materials, but it's worth it. It is very resilient, so it will last through years of use. It conducts body heat and vibration better than other soft materials, and it's much easier to clean. Because it is not porous like other soft materials, you can not only clean it, but you can also disinfect it in a diluted bleach solution (10 parts water to 1 part bleach), by boiling it for about 3 minutes, or by putting it in the top rack of the dishwasher without detergent. Because these toys can be disinfected, they can be shared by different partners. The only drawback is that you cannot use silicone lubricants with them; most silicone lube bonds to a silicone toy and ruins it, so stick to water-based lubes.

Toys made of silicone include dildos, vibrators, butt plugs, wands, cock rings, and penis sleeves. The majority of silicone dildos are designed to be compatible with strap-on harnesses. As the popularity of silicone has grown, some companies have attempted to capitalize on it by using lesser grades of silicone, using a small percentage of silicone, or—worse yet—labeling a toy silicone that's not silicone at all. You want to make sure you purchase toys made of medical-grade or platinum silicone. But unlike other manufacturing industries, the sex toy industry is not regulated by any government agency, so it's not held to any specific standards for what goes into their products, how they're made, or whether they're safe to use. Manufacturers are not required to disclose what a toy is made of on its packaging or elsewhere; furthermore, there is no law against a company printing misleading or incorrect information about what a toy is made of. Still, you can contact toy manufacturers and inquire about what

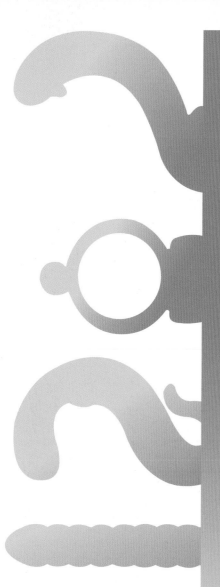

Phthalates Make Toys More Pliable, but at a Cost

Phthalates are added to polyvinyl chloride (PVC) to make it more pliable, so they are often found in soft plastic items, such as toys made for small children, animals, and sexual pleasure. PVC sex toys containing these chemicals are among the most inexpensive and widely available on the market. Although their texture makes them ideal insertables, it turns out that what makes them enjoyable may also make them toxic. Because phthalate-spiked PVC is not a stable, inert compound, these toys continually leach phthalates, which can cause a nasty odor, a greasy film, and, for many people, genital irritation. In studies on mice and rats, high levels of phthalates have been linked to reproductive organ damage, liver damage, and liver cancer; however, there have been no conclusive studies on human beings. There's been enough media coverage about the issue and dialogue among retailers and consumers that many toy manufacturers have begun advertising products as "phthalate-free." If you're concerned about what's in your sex toys, do some research and ask the store where you're buying toys about what materials they are made of.

kind of silicone they use in their toys, or buy toys made by companies with a reputation for top-quality silicone, such as Vixen Creations (which offers a lifetime warranty on its toys), Fun Factory, Tantus Silicone, and Jollies.

Vixen Creations pioneered a special blend of silicone called VixSkin, which marries the best of two worlds: the look and feel similar to materials like CyberSkin with the superior qualities and durability of silicone. VixSkin toys look and feel more realistic than other silicone toys because of the way they are fabricated: They have a firmer inner core that is surrounded by a softer outer layer that mimics the flexibility and softness of real flesh; they are more expensive than regular silicone because they are handmade with a special two-step process.

Hard Plastic and Acrylic: Rock-Hard Toys

Some vibrators and anal toys are made of hard plastic; unlike thermal plastics or rubber-like products, they have no added material to soften them, so they retain a firm, solid texture. Hard plastic is easy to clean, and most toys made of it are less expensive than those made of other materials. Some hard plastic is nonporous and some is not, so always check with the manufacturer. For people who want a firm, inflexible toy without the price tag of glass or metal, hard plastic is a good alternative. However, some hard plastic toys can be expensive, especially if they are made of medical grade, nontoxic plastic.

Acrylic, or Lucite (which is a brand name of acrylic), toys are crystal clear and rock hard; several of the first acrylic toys were designed with dramatic curves especially for the G-spot, including one called the Crystal Wand. Acrylic began to wane in popularity as glass toys appeared, so

there are only a few of these toys left in the marketplace. Like their glass counterparts, acrylic dildos, wands, and butt plugs bring beauty and pleasure together to create works of art that are hypoallergenic, unique, and usually on the expensive side. Well-made acrylic toys should be seamless (seams on a toy reflect lower quality toys that are mass-produced). Their smooth, seamless texture is ideal for penetration, and lube clings to them nicely, too.

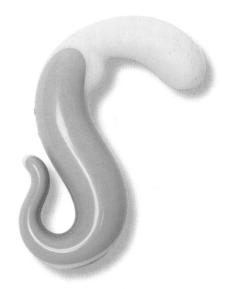

Delight Vibrator

Glass: Like Works of Art, but More Fun

Glass toys (including dildos, double-ended dildos, wands, plugs, and the occasional vibrator) are hard, smooth, and beautiful. Many people consider them works of art in addition to being great sex toys, and many of the designs are simply stunning. Glass lends itself to gorgeous color combinations, interesting textures, and artistic embellishments. If you like firm pressure during penetration, G-spot stimulation, and artistic, hand-crafted toys, then glass may become one of your favorite sex toy materials.

One of the best things about glass is its incredible surface; even the best-quality silicone toy will have some "drag" to it when you run your fingers along it, but not glass. People also like it because it has some weight to it. Glass is seamless and compatible with all kinds of lubricants. Be sure to buy glass toys from a reputable manufacturer and confirm that the toy is made of medical-grade borosilicate or Pyrex, a brand name that has become synonymous with heat- and shock-resistant glass. A properly made borosilicate toy can withstand up to 3,000 pounds of pressure as well as extreme heat and cold.

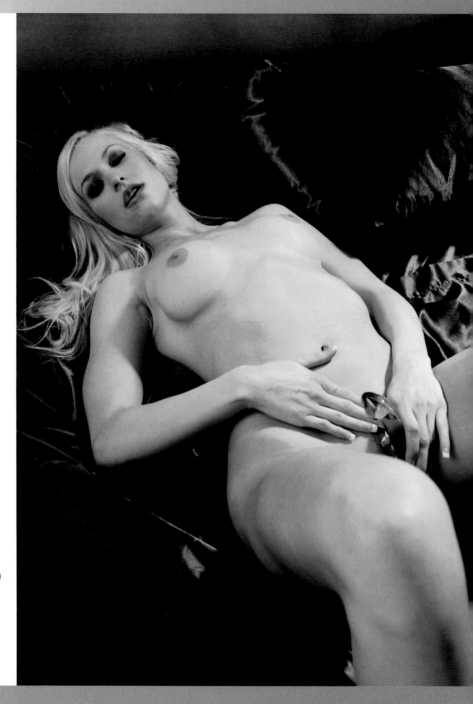

Metal: Smooth, Firm, and Durable

For folks who like a smooth, firm, solid toy, metal toys offer a variety of styles as well as weights. They're durable, are nonporous, and conduct hot and cold temperatures nicely. There are a variety of metal toys on the market, made of aluminum or stainless steel, and some are hollow while others are solid metal. Like glass, these toys create an amazingly smooth sensation for penetration and they hold on to lube well (all lubes work with them). Also like their glass counterparts, metal toys—including dildos, wands, butt plugs, prostate toys, cock rings, and some vibrators—are among the most expensive on the market, but also some of the most beautifully made. Look for metal toys made by one of the top companies: Njoy, Big Teaze, and Tantus Alumina.

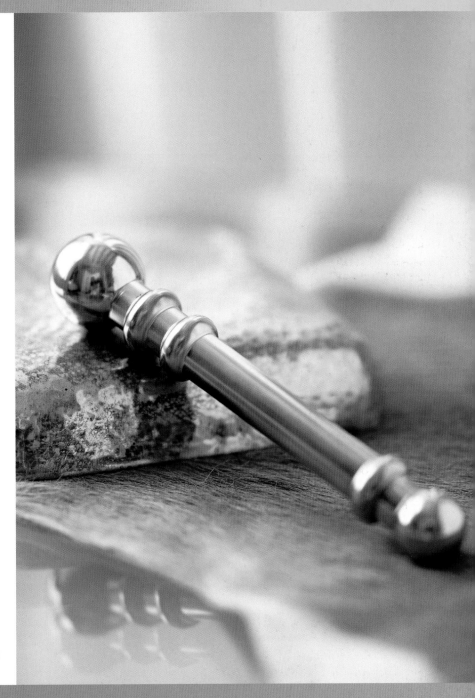

Betty's Vaginal Barbell

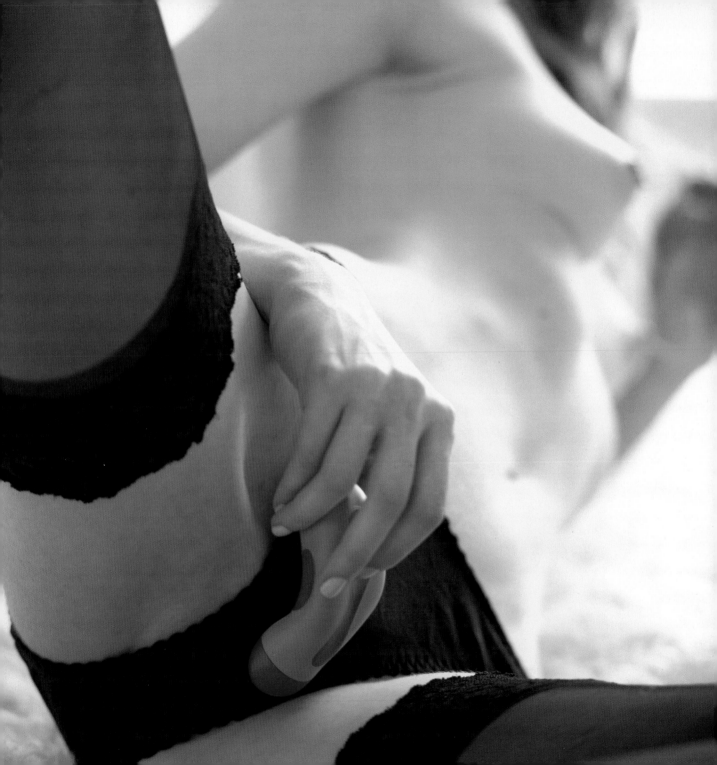

CHAPTER 5
ALL ABOUT VIBRATORS

Vibrators are the most popular of all sex toys on the market, and it's no wonder: When something vibrates against the sensitive genitals or inside the vagina or anus, all the nerve endings come alive. To put it in plain terms: Vibrators feel really good. They can get you in the mood, turn you on, warm you up, make you hot, and get you off.

I cannot tell you how many stories I've heard from women who experienced their very first orgasm by using a vibrator. The truth is that when we begin to masturbate, we're aren't experts right away, and some women find that they can't get the exact technique down to bring themselves to orgasm.

When they try a vibrator, it delivers consistent, focused stimulation that may help them achieve what was once elusive. Many women use vibrators during masturbation to get to know their bodies better, discover what kinds of stimulation they like, and then pass that information on to their partners.

And while it may seem like vibrators are just for women, they aren't! Plenty of men enjoy using vibrating sleeves or pumps and traditional vibrators to stimulate the head of their penis, their balls, or their perineum. Some of the more adventurous ones use vibrators for anal stimulation.

Vibrators aren't just for solo exploration either; they're wonderful for partnered sex. Think of a vibrator as your "extra set of hands" in the bedroom: While you're doing one thing, it can be doing another. Is one hand working her nipples and the other one stroking her hair? A vibrator can be rubbing her vulva when you've got your hands full. Want to spice up oral sex for him? While you've got one hand on his shaft and your lips wrapped around him, slip a vibrator up against his balls. Can't reach to stimulate her clitoris during intercourse in a particular position? Vibrator to the rescue!

For some women, a vibrator can be a big help in getting them aroused. Do you have a low libido? If so, it can take you a long time to get turned on, and you can get frustrated by the process; mentally and emotionally, your desire is red hot, but your body can't catch up. A vibrator can be like a shortcut: It helps to get you relaxed, turned on, and lubricated quicker.

Research shows that the majority of women need clitoral stimulation in order to have an orgasm; it might be clitoral stimulation on its own or combined with penetration, but the clit needs to be in the mix! And we're not talking about any old kind of stimulation. There are plenty of partners who can use their fingers, mouths, tongues or some combination to bring a woman pleasure, but many women need prolonged, targeted stimulation on their clitoris in order to orgasm. Let's face it: People can run out of steam. Their jaws get sore, their necks begin to cramp, and their fingers start to slow down—but a vibrator just keeps on going! And a vibrator can deliver a kind of stimulation no human can, stimulation that's consistent and powerful—the perfect combination of speed, pressure, motion, intensity, and rhythm.

How to Choose a Vibe That Works for You

There is such a wide variety of vibrators on the market that browsing at your local sex shop or online can sometimes be overwhelming. The best place to start is

to decide what you'd like your vibrator to do. Do you want it for external clitoral stimulation only, penetration, or one that can do both? What about a vibrator that's designed for simultaneous penetration and clitoral stimulation? Once you've decided about its function, then you can move on to what you want it to look like. There are insertable vibrators created to look as close to a human penis as possible, with different skin tones, veins, circumcised heads, and sometimes balls. There are others that have a realistic penis-like shape, but come in playful colors like pink, red, green, or purple. Others are designed to resemble something familiar like a tube of lipstick or a cute animal. Some are completely

innocuous looking: small, discreet gadgets most people wouldn't look twice at. Some vibrators are like works of art, with sleek modern shapes, top-of-the-line materials, and satin-lined cases.

You should consider all the elements discussed in chapter 3, including size, cost, and brand and review the different materials covered in chapter 4. Most vibrators are made of rubber, PVC, elastomer, TPR, hard plastic, silicone, or some

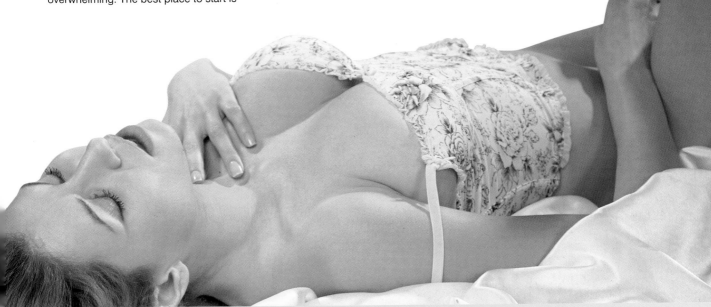

combination. In addition, vibrators are motorized, so they have some specific features to consider. First, what's your speed? Some vibrators have one speed (it's on or it's off); others have a choice of two or three speeds. Some have dials that let you gradually increase or decrease speed, and others have a range from gentle to knock-your-socks-off. As a general rule, battery-powered vibrators have less intense vibration than their plug-in counterparts, and the more batteries, the stronger the intensity. Electric vibrators are considered at the top of the heap for their power, but you need to have an outlet nearby to use them!

In addition to the power and speed of the vibration, many vibrators offer different *types* of vibration. For example, vibes like the Form 6 by Jimmyjane and the SaSi offer different modes, which range in motion from fluttering to undulating to kneading—each of which produces a different sensation. These are the next generation of vibrators that go beyond a one-size-fits-all model and attempt to give you a customized experience.

You may also need to consider how loud a vibrator is, because they range from the whisper quiet kind to the type that sounds like a small appliance running. If you have roommates, thin walls, nosy neighbors, or children, you may want to choose a vibrator on the quieter end of the spectrum. Finally, not all vibrators are waterproof. Those that are will clearly state this feature on the package or in the description; waterproof vibrators are easy to clean (because they can be submerged in water) and are great for people who like to play in the shower, bath, hot tub, or pool.

To give you a better sense of what's available, in the next six chapters, we'll review the different kinds of vibrators, along with their features, how to use them, and some tips for incorporating them into solo and partnered sex. They include:

- Compact clitoral vibrators: small, discreet, battery-powered or rechargeable, designed for external clitoral stimulation, low to moderate vibration; good for beginners, easy to travel with

- Plug-in clitoral vibrators: larger, plug-in, designed for external clitoral stimulation, moderate to intense vibration; unmatched power for those who want strong vibration

- Wearable and hands-free vibrators: unique shapes that you can strap on, sit on, or slip inside during intercourse

- Insertable vibrators: phallic and curved, battery-powered or rechargeable, designed for penetration and G-spot stimulation

- Dual-action vibrators: battery-powered or rechargeable, designed for simultaneous penetration and clitoral stimulation; this group includes "rabbit" vibes

- Smart vibrators: next generation of toys that feature advanced technology, varied features, and top-quality design and materials

- Vibrating cock rings, sleeves, and pumps for men will be featured in later chapters.

OhMiBod and Naughtibod

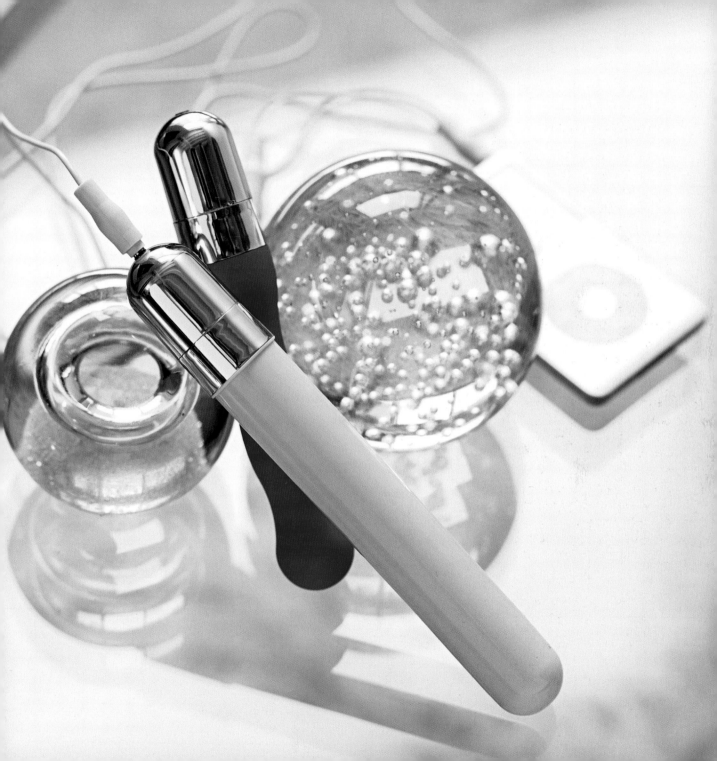

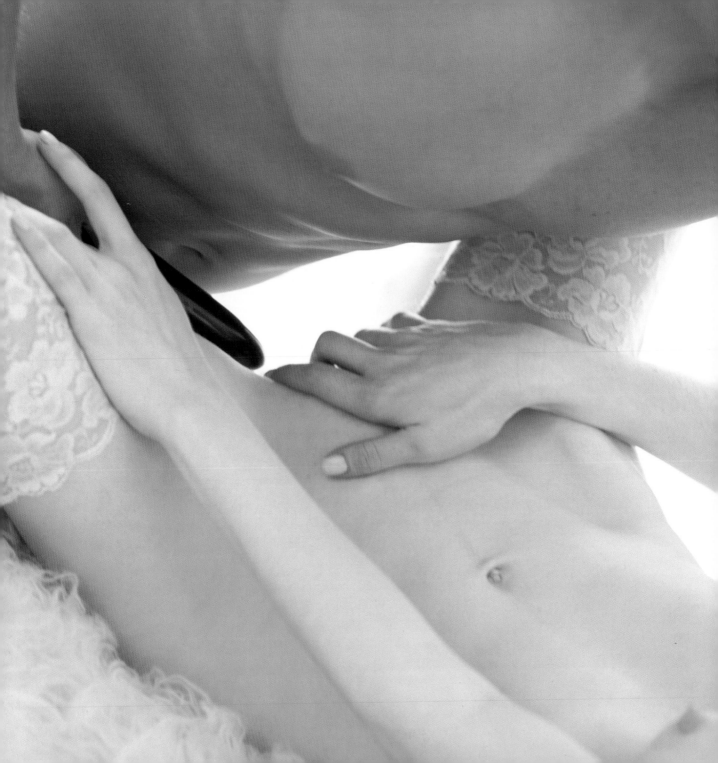

Making a Match:
Tips for Buying Your First Vibrator

Like other "firsts," buying your first vibrator is a big deal!
Reading about all the different kinds of vibrators is a
good step toward discovering what's out there. Next, try
to gather information and advice from some real people.
You can ask your friends about their preferences, visit a
quality sex shop with knowledgeable salespeople, attend
an in-home sex toy party, or read customer reviews of
products on sex toy websites. Look for a vibrator with
multiple speeds, so you can have options. I recommend
choosing one with low to moderate vibration to start out.
If you find you need more power, you can always
upgrade. But, if you start out with something as powerful
as the Hitachi Magic Wand, it may simply be too intense
and may turn you off of the vibrator experience. It's best
to select something inexpensive in case you don't end
up loving it. Save the high-priced luxury vibrators for
when you're sure of what you like.

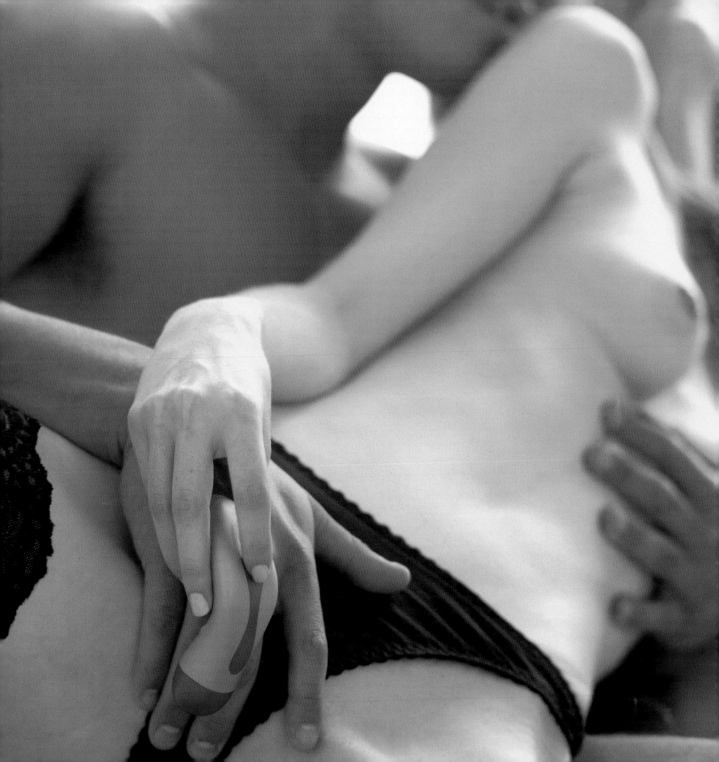

Women's How To: Using a Clitoral Vibrator

They may come with batteries or a stylish carrying case, but most vibrators don't come with instructions! You'll find specific tips in subsequent chapters about using different types of vibrators, but let's start with some basics that apply to all clitoral vibrators. Before you turn it on, you may want to warm yourself up with your own hand or a partner's hand or mouth. In fact, some women like lots of foreplay before a vibrator enters the picture at all because they need to be really aroused. If they aren't warmed up, the stimulation feels way too intense and doesn't feel pleasurable. Some people like to have lots of play, including some intercourse, before reaching for their favorite vibrator. For others, the vibrator is a surefire method to warm up—it's the key to lighting their erotic fire.

Whatever your preference, always begin on a slow speed at first. Be sure to dab some lubricant on the side that comes in contact with your body. Start by placing the vibrator against your inner and outer labia and your vaginal opening. Avoid the clitoris at first as you give your body a chance to rev up. Gradually increase the speed if you want to (and if that's an option). When you're ready, move it to one side of your clitoral hood. You want to approach the clitoris indirectly in the beginning to give yourself a chance to get used to the stimulation. Try each side of the hood, then try the vibrator directly on top of the hood—the hood, not the glans itself. Most women find that a vibrator on top of or to one side of the clitoral hood is plenty stimulating; however, some women like it when you actually pull back the clitoral hood and expose the clitoral glans for direct stimulation. Some women like to do this occasionally or only when they are very, very turned on. Try it and see how it feels for you, and be sure to tell your partner your preference.

If you find the slowest speed of your vibrator too intense even for indirect stimulation, here are a few tricks to decrease the intensity:

- Keep your underwear on while you use the vibrator, so the fabric will slightly mute the vibration.

- Put a washcloth between your vulva and the vibrator; fold it once or twice depending on how much you want to decrease the intensity.

- Place your fingers or hand (or those of your partner) between you and the vibrator; this can diffuse the vibration.

Once you've gotten used to it, you can experiment with different speeds, varying amounts of pressure, and different vibration modes if your vibrator has them. Some people like to move the vibe against them, while others prefer to hold it still and let the vibration itself be the only motion. Whether you are alone or with a partner, explore different positions to find the best ones for you.

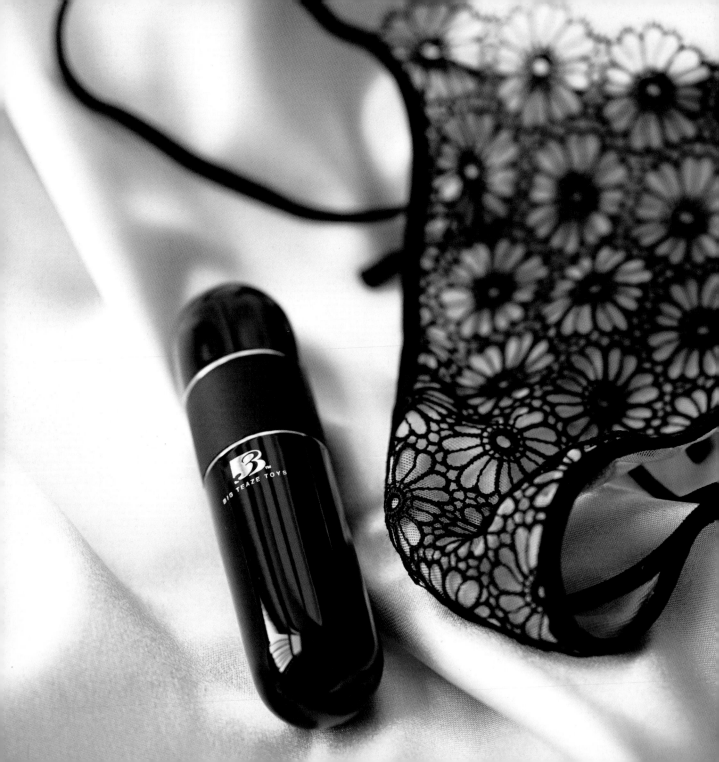

CHAPTER 6

BULLETS, EGGS, AND BUNNIES:

Compact Clitoral Vibrators Create a Buzz

Compact clitoral vibrators are designed for external use against the vulva and clitoris. (They can also be used on nipples, balls, penises, and perineums.) Although they can be used to stimulate the vaginal opening, you should not attempt to use them for penetration. Most of them are compact and discreet, making them ideal for use during intercourse. All of these clitoral vibrators are battery-powered or rechargeable and range from the size of a double A battery to slighter larger than a computer mouse.

Bullets and Eggs: A First-Timer's Delight

Small and portable, bullet-shaped and egg-shaped vibrators are widely available and among the most popular for first-time users. They are usually made of hard plastic and are relatively inexpensive ($10 to $30). The number and type of batteries that power these tiny vibes varies from one watch battery to two or three AA batteries. As a general rule, the more batteries, the greater the intensity. Most egg vibrators are attached with a wire to a separate unit that houses the batteries and features a dial or buttons to control the speed. Some units come with two eggs, so you and your partner can each use one at the same time. Bullet vibes tend to be all-in-one, with one small battery inside the bullet; you turn it on and off and control the speed by twisting a dial on the cap. There are also sleeves sold separately that fit over egg and bullet vibrators; a particular favorite is the bunny, which extends the surface area of the vibrator, conducting the vibration from the body of the rabbit all the way to the ears, which flutter furiously. You'll like these kinds of vibrators if you're a newcomer to the world of vibration, you like low to moderate intensity, or you're shy about using a vibrator.

Can I Get Addicted to My Vibrator?

This is one of the most common questions I get asked, and it's something a lot of people are concerned about. First, people worry that once they learn to reach orgasm with a vibrator and get used to it, they'll never be able to go back to the old days: They won't be able to come with their hands, their lover's fingers, or oral sex. Not true! Sure, you can definitely grow accustomed to climaxing with the help of a vibrator, just as you can get used to coming in a certain position. If this concerns you, then simply switch it up from time to time, and practice having an orgasm in many different ways so you don't get hung up on just one. Second, people think that vibrators can desensitize, numb, or damage the clitoris—which is also untrue. Can you overdo it? Of course. Just like with lots of other things, moderation is best. If you use your vibrator for hours of multiple orgasms, your clitoris may feel overly sensitive, worn out, sore, or even numb. Don't worry, the feeling isn't permanent. Give your body a break and a chance to recover, and it will be back to itself in no time.

Tristan's Top Pick: Bullet

The Onyé by Big Teaze Toys is a stainless steel and silicone bullet that's compact, quiet, and simply stunning. Like Goldilocks, if you've been searching for a vibrator that's more intense than other bullets but not too intense, you may find that the Onyé is just right! Remember, though, that luxury comes with a price: This is one of the most expensive bullets on the market ($55 to $65).

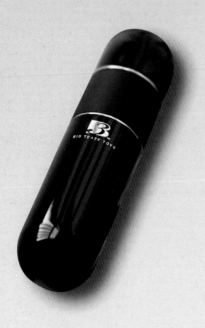

Fingertip Vibes: Give Your Digits a Helping Hand

Because many women first learn to stimulate their clitoris with their hands, it seems fitting that there's a style of vibrator created to give your fingers a helping hand! Although plenty of women say that fingers (their own or their partner's) can produce the perfect stimulation, why not add a little buzz to those already award-worthy techniques? Made of hard plastic and rubber or silicone, fingertip vibes slide right over the fingertip like a ring and feature a small on/off switch on one side (and are usually under $30). They're great if you are looking to intensify your finger's power or take over when your digits need a break. This kind of vibe works equally well for solo or partnered adventures and is extremely quiet. They are good for beginners because the speed is low to moderate.

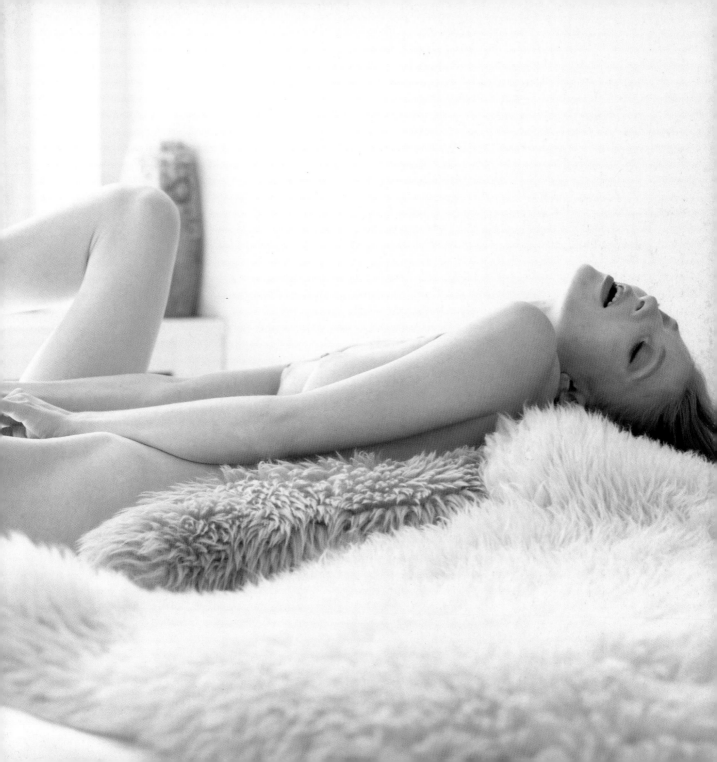

You're Worth the Splurge: Luxury Compact Clitoral Vibrator

Imagine that a bullet vibrator were stretched out to be more than 5 inches (13 cm) long and had no separate control unit, and you've got the Little Something vibrator made by luxury manufacturer/retailer Jimmyjane. It's got the perks of the best compact vibes: It's waterproof, is whisper quiet, and runs on one battery. And, of course, it's small and discreet enough to leave out on the nightstand, throw in your purse, or travel with. But here's what makes it luxury: It's available in 24K gold or platinum ($325 to $3,250)!

Pocket Rocket: Discreet Design, Powerful Buzz

Band-Aid is such a well-known brand that it has become synonymous with adhesive bandages. Similarly, the Pocket Rocket is thought of not just as a brand name but also as a particular style of compact vibrator. About the size of a lipstick, only slightly taller, it is made of hard plastic and runs on one double A battery, which sits in the lower two-thirds of the vibrator. You twist the base to turn it on and off (and to open it to replace the battery). It has a rounded top with several metal nubs on it; this texture feels really good against the vulva and clitoris. Some pocket rocket vibes are also sold with plastic caps with different bumps and ridges, and most are under $30. Leaving the cap on can not only change the top's texture but also slightly mute the intensity of the vibration. This kind of vibrator looks completely innocuous to your spying roommate or the TSA inspector at the airport. There is only one speed, but it's more powerful than many of the other vibrators in this chapter. There is also a mini version (which is about half the size) and a waterproof version called the Water Dancer.

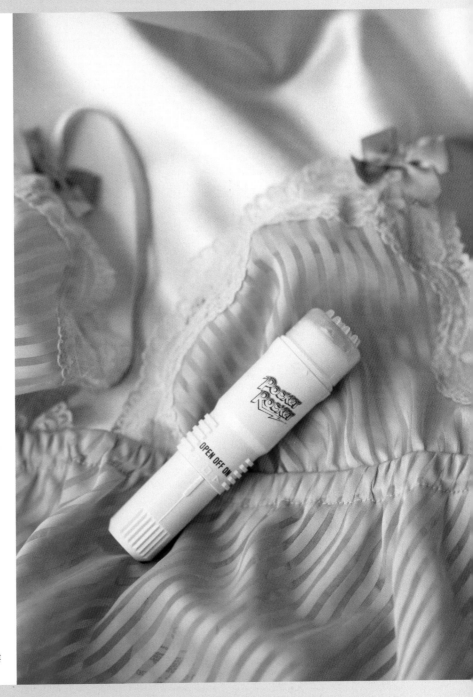

Pocket Rocket

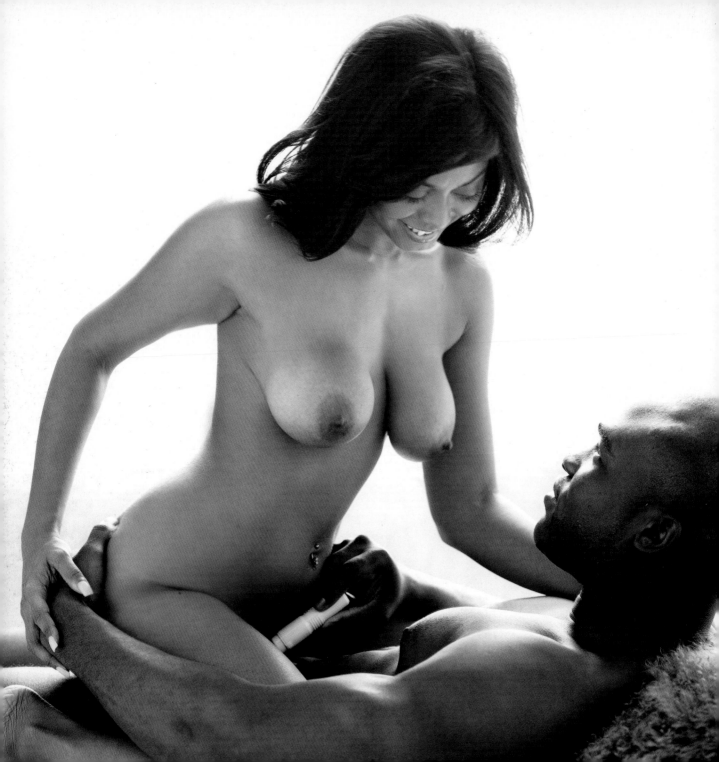

Perfect Pairing: Finger Vibe or Pocket Rocket + Cowgirl Position

In the Cowgirl position, he lays on his back with his legs together, and she sits on top and faces him. She can control the angle, depth, and rhythm of the penetration, and he can lie back and let her take charge. Not only does he have a wonderful view of her body and the penetration action, but he also has easy access to her clitoris. Whether he slips on a finger vibe or grabs a pocket rocket, he can hold the vibrator against her clitoris as she moves on top of him. If she wants more pressure against her clitoris, she can lean forward toward him. If she wants less intense vibration but there is only one speed option on the vibrator, he can put his finger (or she can put her own finger) between her clitoris and the vibrator. This will decrease the intensity of the stimulation.

Disguised Vibes: They May Look Innocent But . . .

Lots of different kinds of vibrators fit into this category, but they all have one thing in common: They're disguised as something else. Some disguised vibes are very small, making them easy to slip into a purse, take on a weekend getaway, or use during intercourse with a partner. The Lipstick Vibrator ($30) is the perfect choice for a girl on the go who likes to be discreet; it looks exactly like an indispensable makeup tool—a perfect disguise if it falls out of your handbag onto a stranger's lap at the coffee shop! There's also a vibe that looks like a pen and one whose case looks like a roll of hard candy. For those of you who like their vibes to be as cute as they are reliable, look for one of the many small vibrators that resemble cuddly animals such as bunnies, ducks, bears, and beavers; these are usually made of rubber and contain an egg or bullet vibrator within the body of the animal.

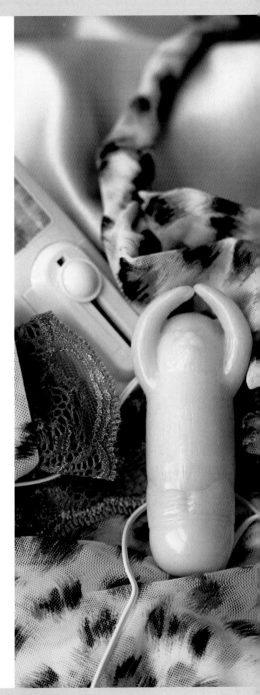

The Honey Bear

You're Worth the Splurge: Luxury Ergonomic Clitoral Vibrators

The Pebble (available at Myla, $165) is a hard plastic vibrator designed by Japanese sculptural ceramicist Mari-Ruth Oda. Its shape is truly unique: It resembles a large rock with ergonomic indents meant to fit perfectly against a woman's vulva and clitoris. It's rechargeable and a perfect gift for the nature girl in your life.

Lelo is a luxury toy maker based in Sweden that produces some of the most stunning toy designs on the market. The Yva ($1,500) is an 18K-gold-plated compact vibe that is quiet, rechargeable, and beautifully packaged.

Solo Play for Her: Honey Bear by Vibratex

Don't be deceived by its adorable appearance: The Honey Bear ($20) means business and makes a great toy for masturbation. Lying on your back, place the well-lubed bear against your vulva with its head and paws below the clitoris and turn it on at the lowest speed. Let it vibrate against your inner labia and vaginal opening to begin the arousal process; avoid direct stimulation of your clitoris in the beginning. As you feel yourself start to get more turned on, gradually inch the bear up until the paws are on either side of the clitoral hood and the bear's head is directly on top of the hood. Experiment with changing the speed of the vibration and see how your body responds. Also try applying different amount of pressure against the vibrator to see what works best for you. Think about what types of oral or manual stimulation you like to determine how to use the vibrator to suit you best. For example, if you like a light flick of the tongue against your clitoris, you want to apply light pressure. If you prefer to rub your clit hard, try pressing the vibrator firmly against you.

Ergonomic Vibes Hug Your Curves in All the Right Places

Imagine a sleek, streamlined computer mouse that has been modified to mimic the curves of a woman's pelvic area. That's the general aesthetic of ergonomic vibrators, which are made of hard plastic or hard plastic covered in silicone. For women looking for a vibrator that does not remotely resemble either a penis or an animal or one whose form is as cool as its function, ergonomic vibes provide a great sense of style along with solid performance. These vibrators are designed to hug a woman's curves, so they are great for both solo and partner play. If you like a fast tongue against your clitoris or quick but gentle fingers rubbing it, then an ergonomic vibrator is a good choice for you. Some of the most popular in this category are:

- Superbe by Natural Contours ($20 to $25): one of the first ergonomic styles on the market; compact vibrator features three different speeds and a discreet look

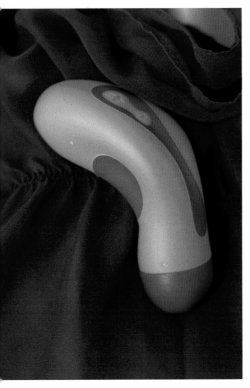

Laya Spot

- Laya Spot by Fun Factory ($40 to $50): a silicone powerhouse with a perfect shape and a good speed range from low to high

- Nea by Lelo ($85 to $95): a gorgeous, expensive design masterpiece with moderate vibration that's rechargeable

Perfect Pairing: Laya Spot + Missionary L Position

In Missionary L position, she lies on her back and he kneels between her legs. He raises her legs so they are perpendicular to her body and one ankle rests on each of his shoulders. This position is different from traditional Missionary in two important ways: It allows for deeper penetration and it gives both of you more access to her clitoris. She can slide an ergonomic vibrator in between her legs and hold it there as he thrusts in and out of her. The vibrator's compact design means it won't get in the way of his thrusting and she can easily adjust the speed.

Tristan's Top Picks

Bullet: Pipedream Luv Touch Bullet Vibe ($20 to $25)

Fingertip: Fukuoku 9000 ($25 to $30)

Pocket rocket: Water Dancer by Vibratex ($20 to $30)

Disguise: Incognito Lipstick Vibrator by Topco Grrl Toyz ($25 to $30)

Ergonomic: Laya Spot by Fun Factory ($40 to $50)

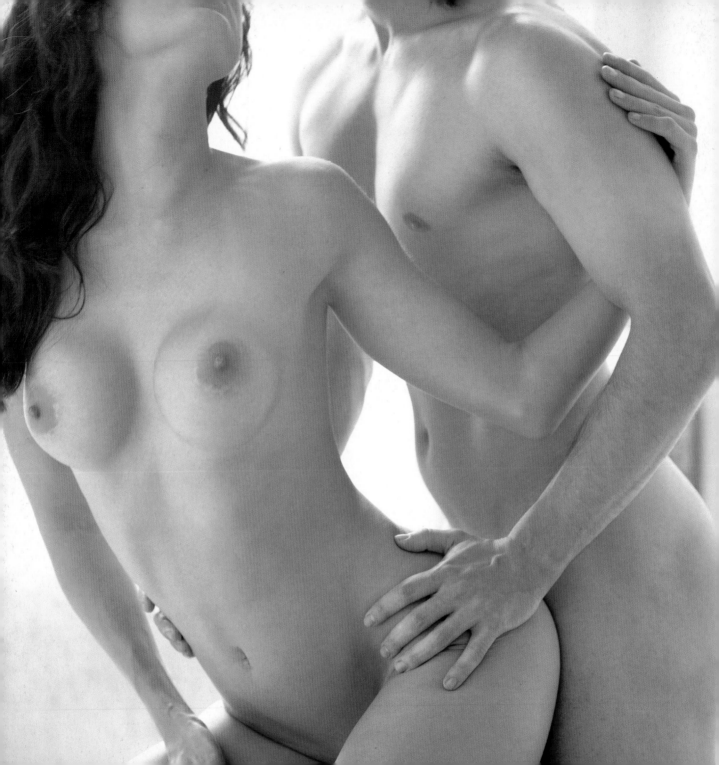

CHAPTER 7

POWER UP:

Clitoral Vibrators Boost the Buzz

When they were first invented and prescribed for women to cure various kinds of ailments, all vibrators were electric. Today, the majority of vibrators are battery-powered, but electric vibrators remain very popular for one important reason: their power. If you find that battery-powered vibrators don't offer a strong enough sensation, fast enough vibration, or intense enough experience, then you may want to consider an electric vibrator. These plug-in wonders just cannot be beat when it comes to intensity. Electric vibrators come in several different styles, including wand style (both plug in and rechargeable), coil-powered, and oscillating. All the vibrators in this chapter are used for external clitoral stimulation only.

Hitachi Magic Wand: A Best Seller, but Not for Newbies

The Hitachi Magic Wand ($50 to $60) first hit store shelves in the 1970s, when physicians began recommending it as a muscle massager. Soon after, women discovered it worked well as a clitoral vibrator, and it's been a runaway success ever since. A best-selling vibrator at toy stores all over the country, the Magic Wand is considered to be the cream of the crop of plug-in, wand-style vibrators. It is the most powerful vibrator on the market today, and thousands of women swear there simply is nothing like their Magic Wand. The Hitachi Magic Wand has a body the size of a paper towel roll (just the roll, without the paper towels) and a flexible, cushiony plastic head the size of a tennis ball (although the head is not completely round; it's more similar to the shape of a marshmallow).

When I worked at sex-positive store Babeland in New York, women used to come in and ask for the Hitachi Magic Wand by name, often because a friend of theirs raved about it. I asked them about their experience level, because the Hitachi is not necessarily the best choice for a first vibrator. Even its lower speed is quite intense, and it may simply be *too* intense for some women, especially newcomers to the world of clitoral vibrators. If you're not quite sure yet what kind of vibrator you want, you may want to try something with batteries first.

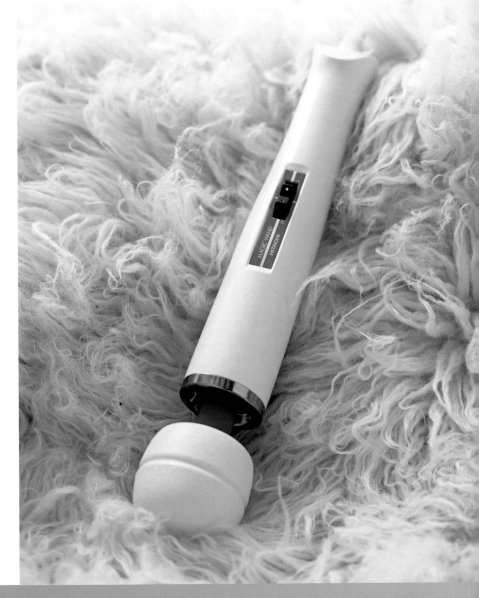

The Magic Wand has two speeds, low and high, and both are strong, fast, and intense. To use this kind of vibrator, hold onto the body and press the head against your clit. Because of its size, the head can cover a lot of surface area. If you like the feeling of vibration against your vulva, then press the head so that it covers both the clitoral hood and the inner labia. If you want the vibration to be concentrated on your clit, you can hold the vibrator so that the edge of the head sits on top of the clitoral hood. If you prefer a specific side of your clitoris, hold the vibrator's head against that side.

If you find that the vibration is just too intense for you, see my tips for decreasing the intensity on page 57. Although its imposing size may intimidate some people, don't be fooled; even though it's much larger than the compact vibrators in the previous chapter, you can still use it during intercourse in most, but not all, positions. To use it in Missionary position, have him sit up between your legs rather than lie down on top of you. Either one of you can hold the vibrator in this position. You'll have plenty of room for the vibrator in all the woman-on-top positions, including Cowgirl and Reverse Cowgirl. You can hold the vibrator yourself in Doggie Style and its variations. Because of its large head and strong vibration, often your partner will be able to feel the vibration against his shaft or balls in many positions, which is an added bonus.

The Magic Wand was designed for external clitoral stimulation, but some folks wish that they could harness all that power and intensity in an insertable toy. The Gee Whiz by Vixen Creations ($50) is a silicone attachment that fits nicely over the head of the Magic Wand and transforms it into a G-spot vibrator.

Perfect Pairing: Hitachi Magic Wand + Spoon Position

In Spoon position, she lies on her side and he lies behind her and enters her from behind. She can also swing one leg over his leg to give him better access to her vagina and anus. This position gives partners a lot of skin-to-skin contact and closeness, although no face-to-face communication or eye contact. It also does not allow for deep or powerful thrusting, making it an ideal position for a man with a long penis or a woman who likes more shallow penetration. Spoon position works very well with vaginal or anal intercourse and the Hitachi Magic Wand, because the vibrator won't get in the way of his thrusting. Her vulva and clitoris are completely accessible, and she can move the vibrator around to find the perfect spot for it. This position also works well because she does not have to hold herself up in any way, since many women like to hold the Magic Wand with both hands.

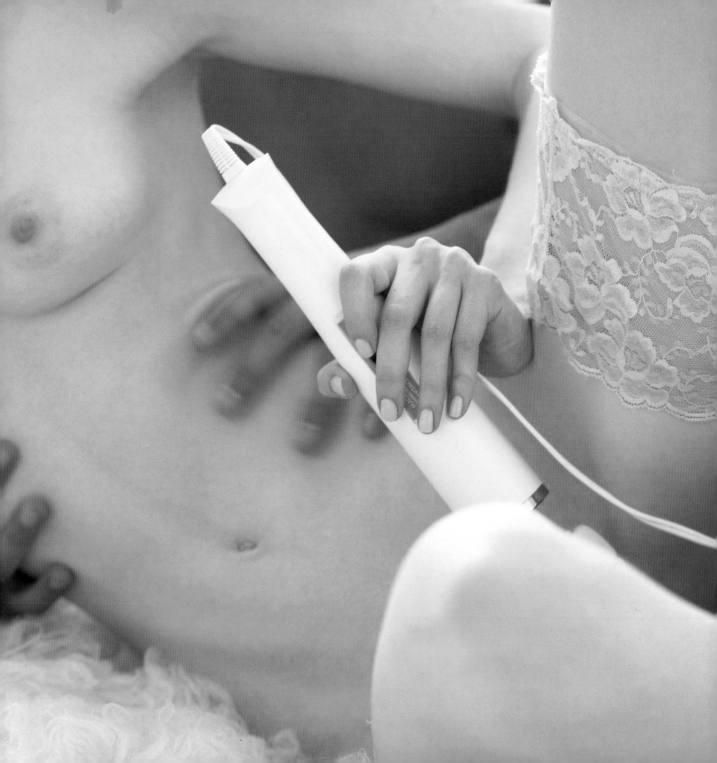

Unplug with Wand-Style Rechargeables

For people who like the style of the Magic Wand but don't want to bother with extension cords or always having an outlet nearby, there are several wand-style rechargeable vibrators. Although these kinds of vibrators are pretty powerful, you will sacrifice some intensity for convenience. The Acuvibe ($75 to $80) resembles the Magic Wand most closely, and it is also the most powerful of the rechargeable wands. It has a flexible, soft head that is about 2 inches (5 cm) wide, providing plenty of surface area; the vibration is concentrated in the head, rather than spread throughout the entire massager. When fully charged, it works for about 45 minutes. The Wahl 2-Speed Rechargeable Massager ($30 to $40) also looks a lot like the Magic Wand except its flexible, cushiony head is surrounded by a ring of raised bumps, adding texture to the vibration; if you like pressure against your clitoris during masturbation or you prefer textured, nubby toys, then you'll like the Wahl. It needs to be charged for 45 minutes, and will hold a charge for about a half hour. Natural Contours' Ideal

vibrator ($60) has a similar look except that the head is smooth and soft and the wand part is bent, which some people find easier to grip and maneuver. If you find the other styles too bulky, you may prefer the Ideal. After 4 hours of charging time, it can last for up to an hour and a half.

Perfect Pairing: Acuvibe + Doggie-Style Position

In Doggie-Style position, she gets on her hands and knees and he enters her from behind. Because this position is rear-entry, there is plenty of room for a larger vibrator; plus, with the Acuvibe, you don't have to fuss with cords or plugging it in. Wrap your hand around the vibrator and hold it so that it's parallel with your torso. Press the head either above the clitoral hood (for less direct, intense stimulation) or directly over the hood (for more intense stimulation). As he thrusts, use your other hand for balance. If this gets to be too difficult, try putting your head and shoulders down so that you're leaning on top of the vibrator; this way, you won't get tired from trying to balance and hold the vibrator at the same time.

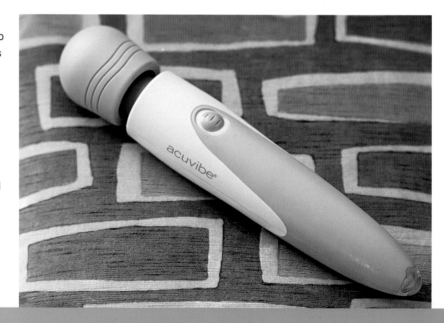

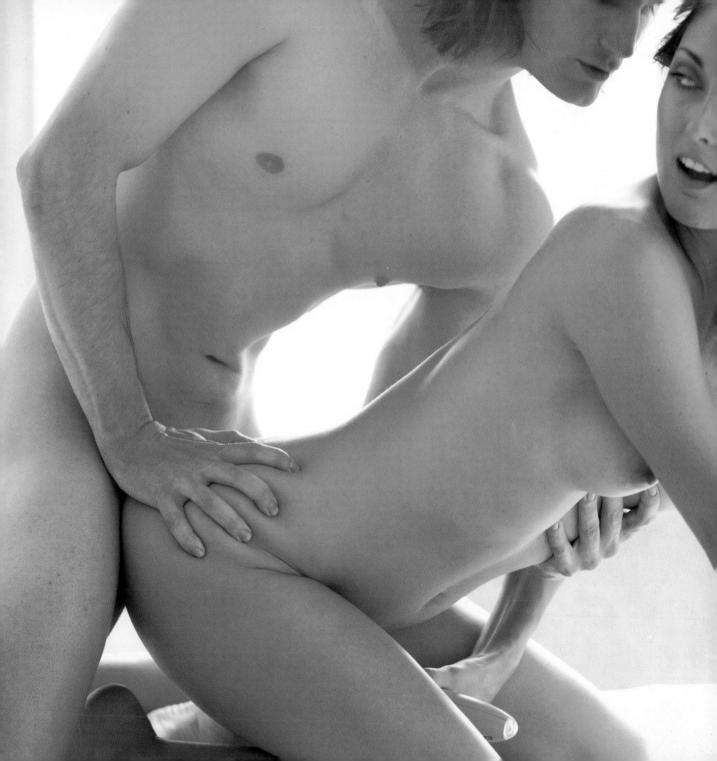

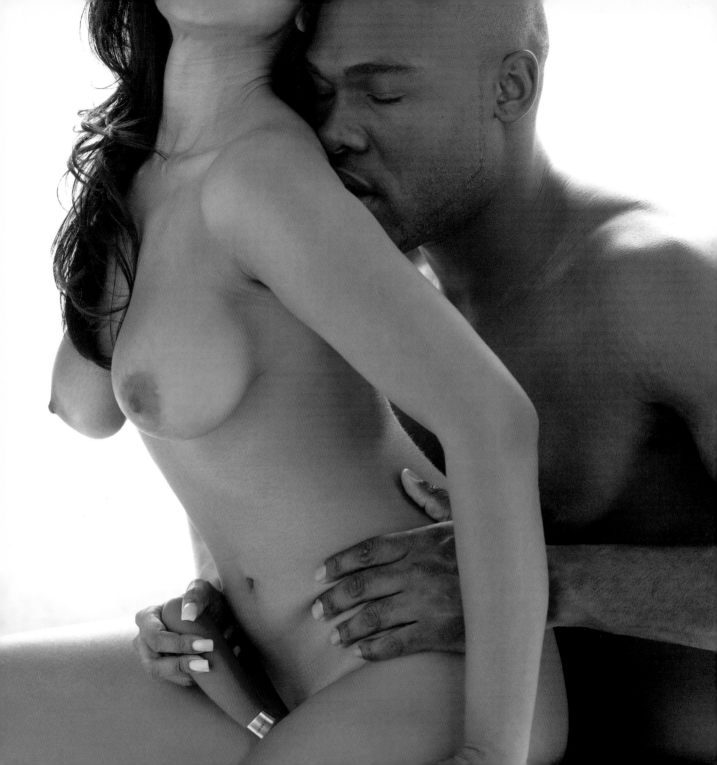

Wahl 7-in-1: Quiet, but Powerful

It may look like a vibrator from decades ago, and some say it resembles a handheld electric mixer, but don't let its less-than-stylish appearance fool you! The Wahl 7-in-1 coil vibrator ($40) is a versatile, powerful toy. Like the Hitachi Magic Wand, the Wahl was originally introduced as a "personal massager" for sore muscles, but quickly developed a following of women who discovered it worked a lot better between their legs. Whereas most vibrators have a motor that produces their vibration, the Wahl 7-in-1 features an electromagnetic coil that the tip of the vibrator vibrates against at about 60 times per second. The coil means that this is one of the quietest vibes on the market and definitely the quietest of all plug-ins, so if you have roommates, nosy neighbors, or thin walls, then you may want to consider it. This toy features two speeds and some of the fastest vibration of any vibrator; many women say that it provides more focused stimulation than the Magic Wand. If you find that the Magic Wand feels too powerful or seems like it's going to numb your clit rather than make it sing, try the Wahl. It comes with seven different attachments—each with a different shape and texture.

Eroscillator: An Entirely Different Experience

If you're looking for the power of a plug-in vibrator but want a gentler motion against your clitoris, you can try the Eroscillator ($130 to $250). The Eroscillator is an entirely unique vibrator; it looks and works differently than any other electric vibe. Most electric vibrators contain a rotational motor; when you turn them on, the motor moves rapidly in a circle, which creates the vibration, and it usually vibrates either the entire toy or concentrates vibration in the head or tip of it. This design creates a steady, powerful kind of pounding motion, which works for many women, but doesn't for others. In the Eroscillator, the motor oscillates—moves back and forth very quickly (about 3,600 oscillations per minute)—instead of rotates, and the attachment is connected directly to the motor; all of this creates a different kind of motion than other vibrators. Think about how you prefer oral sex: Do you like your partner to move his tongue back and forth quickly or do you like a circular motion? If you like the back-and-forth motion or if you've tried electric vibrators in the past and found the vibration to be too "thuddy" or overwhelming, then you may prefer an oscillating vibrator like the Eroscillator.

The Eroscillator is sold in different packages: The basic Eroscillator 2 comes with three different heads, or you can buy one of several deluxe versions that come with up to seven different heads. Each head has a different shape and texture. Another major difference to consider: The attachment heads for the Eroscillator are much smaller (about the size of a quarter) than the heads of electric wand vibrators. So, if you like a large head with plenty of surface area, the Eroscillator probably won't meet your needs.

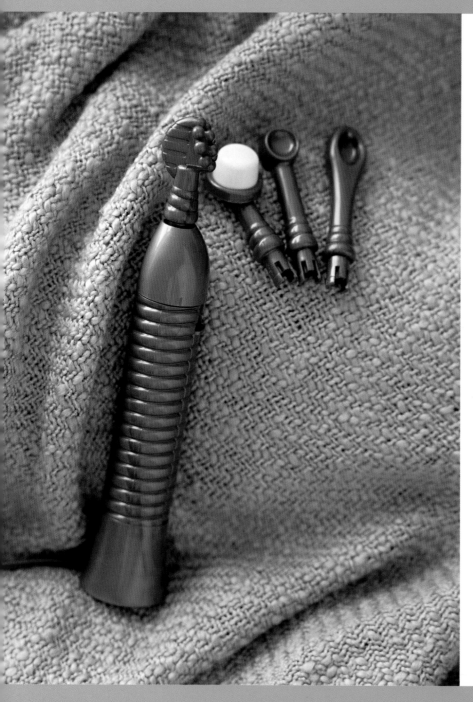

Perfect Pairing: Eroscillator + Lap Dance Position

In the Lap Dance position, he sits in a chair with his legs together and she straddles him with her legs apart facing away from him. Pick a simple chair rather than an overstuffed one with large arms, and make sure your feet can touch the ground. The woman is firmly in charge of this position and can take control of the angle of penetration, the depth, the speed, and the overall rhythm. She can use her legs and feet for leverage and also push off his thighs with her hands. He can reach around and hold the Eroscillator's head against her clitoris as she rides him.

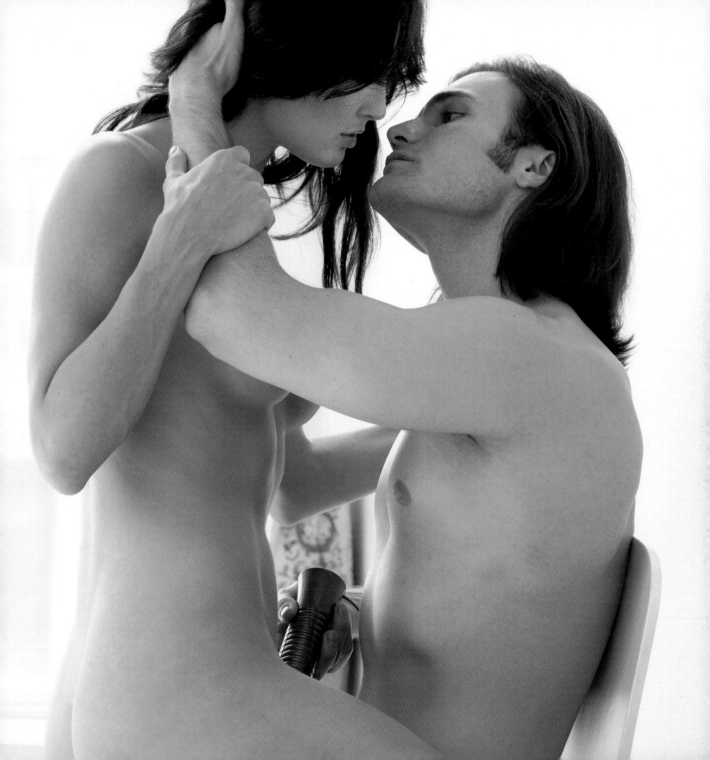

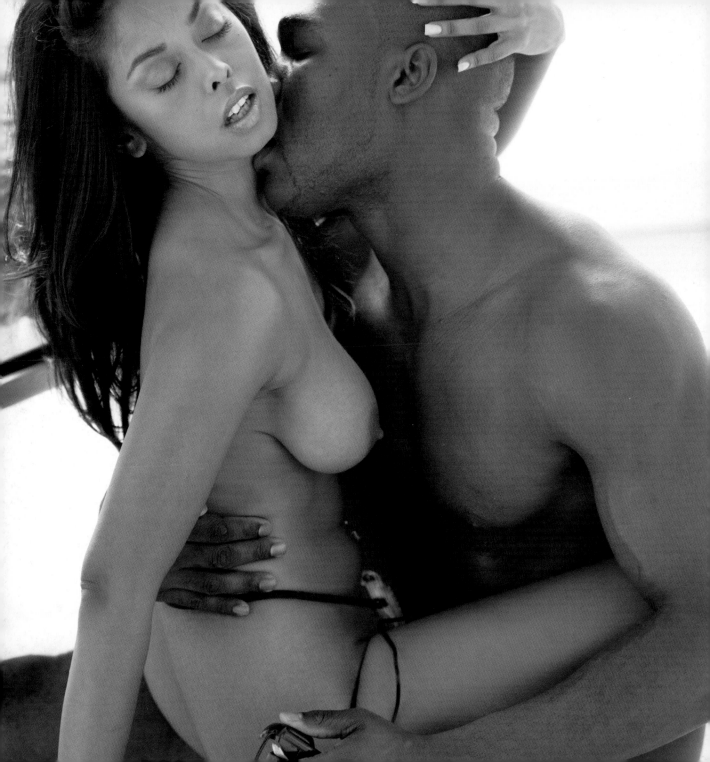

CHAPTER 8

LOOK MA, NO HANDS:

Wearable Vibrators

As you cup his balls and run your nails up and down his chest, he plays with your inner labia and rolls your nipples around between his fingers, suddenly, the dilemma is clear: Who's going to hold the vibrator? When using a vibrator during partnered sex, it's often true that you don't have an extra hand to spare. Wearable and hands-free vibrators are a great solution to this problem! These vibrators—some for external clitoral stimulation, others for both external and internal stimulation—free up your hands to do other things while working their vibrating magic on your most sensitive parts.

Wearable Clitoral Vibes

Wearable vibrators ($20 to $50) do just what their name indicates: They are small vibrators attached to elastic straps that fit around your hips and thighs, so you can actually wear the vibrator. Most of them are designed to resemble something in nature, such as dolphins, flowers, or butterflies. If you like positions where you are facing each other with lots of skin-to-skin contact—such as Missionary, Straddle, and Missionary CAT—they often leave little room for a vibrator or even your hand to slip between your legs. Wearable vibes are great to use during intercourse in these positions. To use this kind of vibe, step into the straps like a pair of panties, then pull it up and position the vibrator so that it's right where you want it. Tighten and adjust the straps so they feel snug against you. Wearable vibrators are designed with intercourse in mind, so none of the straps should be blocking your vagina or anus. Once it feels good, you're free to play with his hair, hold his face, tweak his nipples, and wrap your arms around him.

Keep in mind that there are a few downsides to wearable vibes. No matter which brand you get, universally, the vibration tends to be low to medium. Remember, these are small and battery-powered, and you sacrifice power for the convenience and novelty of a hands-free experience. One of the biggest complaints I heard from women while working at Babeland was that the vibration was just too weak to really get them going. But that won't be a problem for you if you already use a battery-powered vibe and it works fine for you. Another issue is that they aren't always well made; the straps often stretch out and don't always stay in place, meaning you have to reach down and hold the vibe where you want it—thus defeating its primary purpose of being hands-free!

If you like the idea of a hands-free experience, but don't want to use the vibe for intercourse, then consider trying a pair of vibrating panties. Vibrating panties are fun little items that come in a variety of different fabrics and styles, from satin and crotchless to latex or lacy. The panty usually has a built-in pocket or pouch to hold a removable vibrator. They may not work for intercourse, but they are great for masturbation or to wear out on a date where no one knows you have them on. If you pick vibrating panties with a remote control, your partner can carry the remote while you are at the mercy of his button pushing.

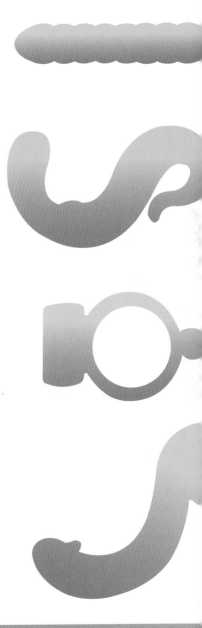

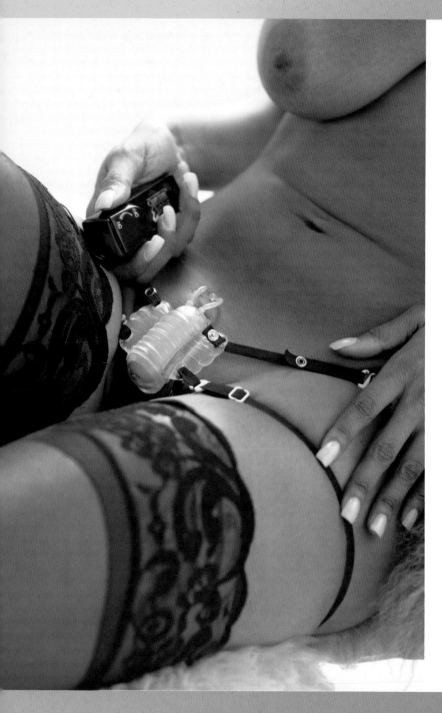

Perfect Pairing: Dolphin Vibe + Yab-Yum Position

Yab-Yum is a classic Tantric sex position where one partner sits in the other partner's lap and they face each other. The woman should strap on the Dolphin wearable vibrator ($35 to $40) before they get into the position. The man sits with his legs loosely crossed and the woman sits in his lap and wraps her legs around his waist and torso. He can use firm pillows under his thighs if he needs more support for his legs. If it's not comfortable for him to keep his legs crossed, then he can stretch them out in front of him. If he needs back support, he can lean against the wall or headboard. As she gets into his lap, she can rise up slightly on her knees, and he can hold the base of his penis to assist her, and she can slowly come down onto it. This is meant to be a relaxing, meditative position, so once you're in it, you shouldn't feel any tension or strain. If you do, adjust yourselves so that you can comfortably sink into the position. Look into each other's eyes, and take advantage of the closeness this position affords you. Because there is so much skin-to-skin contact, there isn't a lot of room for a vibrator or even to slip a hand between her legs to stimulate her

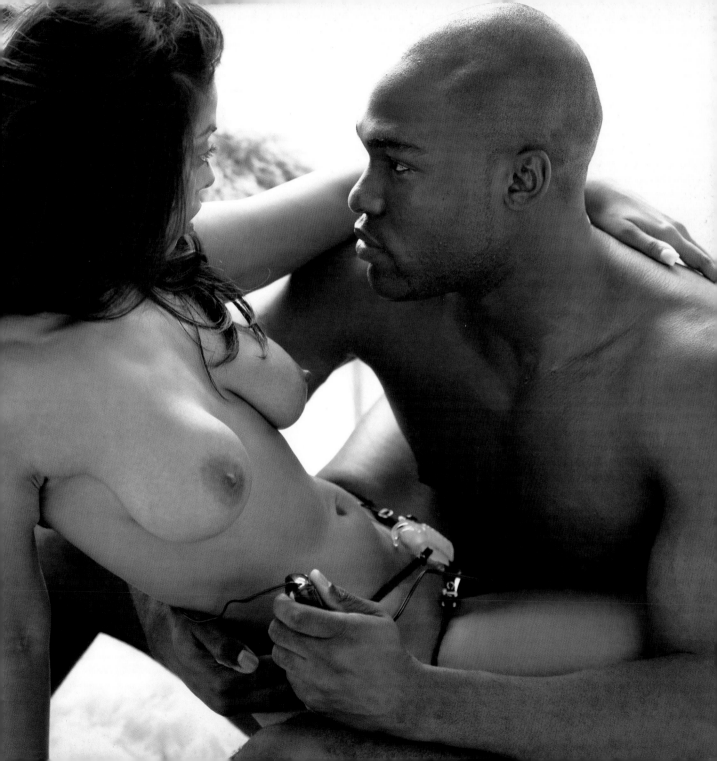

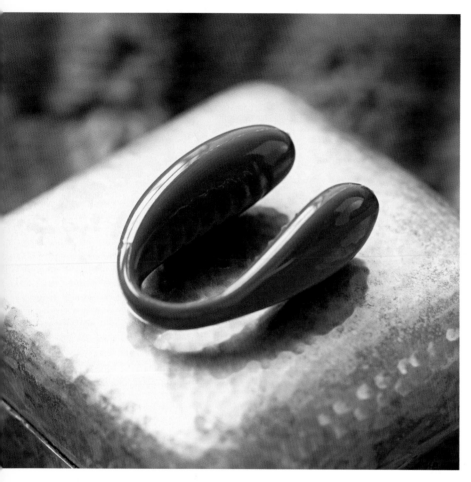

clitoris. The Dolphin vibe is perfect for Yab-Yum: It can nestle against her clit, buzzing quietly, as you experience slow, rocking, gentle thrusting.

Hands-Free Insertable Vibes

The original and best product in this category is the We-Vibe ($130), a silicone, rechargeable, waterproof vibrator that delivers simultaneous clitoral and G-spot stimulation. The We-Vibe is U-shaped and resembles a soft pair of tongs with one slimmer end and one wider end. One of the great things about the We-Vibe is that it's so slim that you can wear it during intercourse, and it doesn't get in the way of penetration; in fact, it was designed to be used during penetration. Slide the slimmer end inside the vagina and as you do so, the wider end hugs the entire vulva. With every thrust of your partner's fingers, dildo, or penis, the internal portion rubs and vibrates right against the G-spot, while the wider, external end vibrates against the clitoris. Because it's so slim, most men don't feel like it's in the way during intercourse, although they do feel the vibration—which is a good thing!

Although it was designed for hands-free external and internal pleasure during intercourse, women can also wear the We-Vibe for hands-free masturbation as well. Versatile and flexible, it's a great vibrator for men, too! Try putting it around the base of his penis and closing the two ends together. Or turn it around and let it cradle (and stimulate) his balls. You can also rub it against the sensitive frenulum on the underside of the penis.

Perfect Pairing: We-Vibe + Horizontal Tailgate Position

In Horizontal Tailgate position, she lies on her stomach with her legs together, and he lies almost completely on top of her. This is a very intimate position; it's got many of the pros of Doggie Style with more skin-to-skin contact and closeness. However, one of the challenges of Horizontal Tailgate is that it's quite difficult for either of you to reach and stimulate her clitoris when she's lying on her stomach. With the We-Vibe, you can easily achieve hands-free clitoral stimulation in this position. Begin with her in a traditional Doggie-Style position and you kneeling behind her. Slide the well-lubricated slimmer end of the We-Vibe inside her vagina; press your hand against the wider side that rests against her clitoris to give her some added pressure to the vibration. Slide a finger inside her vagina and press against the vibrator. When she's ready, slowly enter her from behind; she can part her legs or tip her hips slightly up toward you to make the initial insertion easier. Once you're inside her, lean all the way forward so that you're lying on top of her. Unlike Doggie Style, you can't do a lot of deep or powerful thrusting in Horizontal Tailgate; instead, aim to make small rocking movements and take advantage of the closeness this position affords you to kiss the back of her neck, whisper in her ear, and stroke her hair. As you move inside her, the We-Vibe vibrates both internally and externally, working her G-spot and clitoris at the same time. This one is definitely a recipe for multiple orgasms!

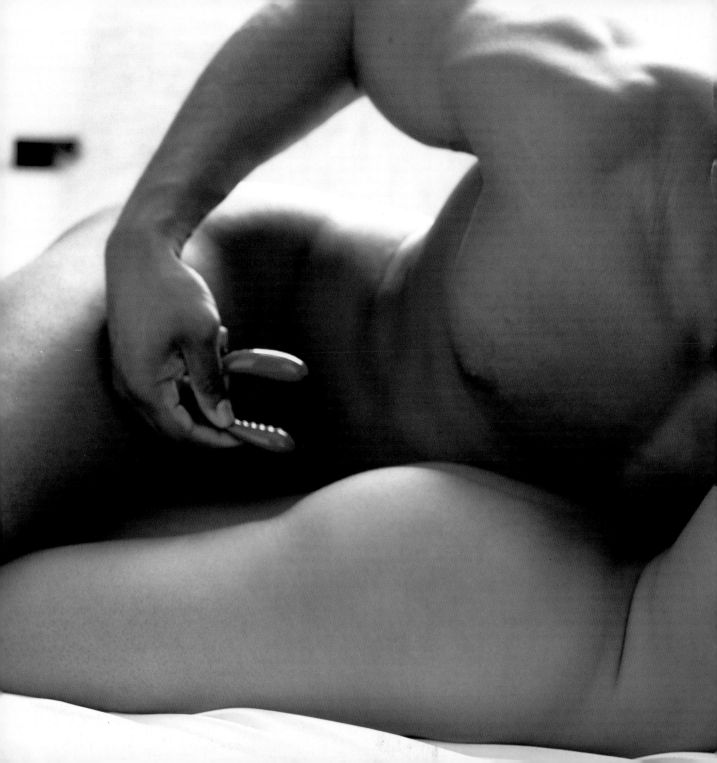

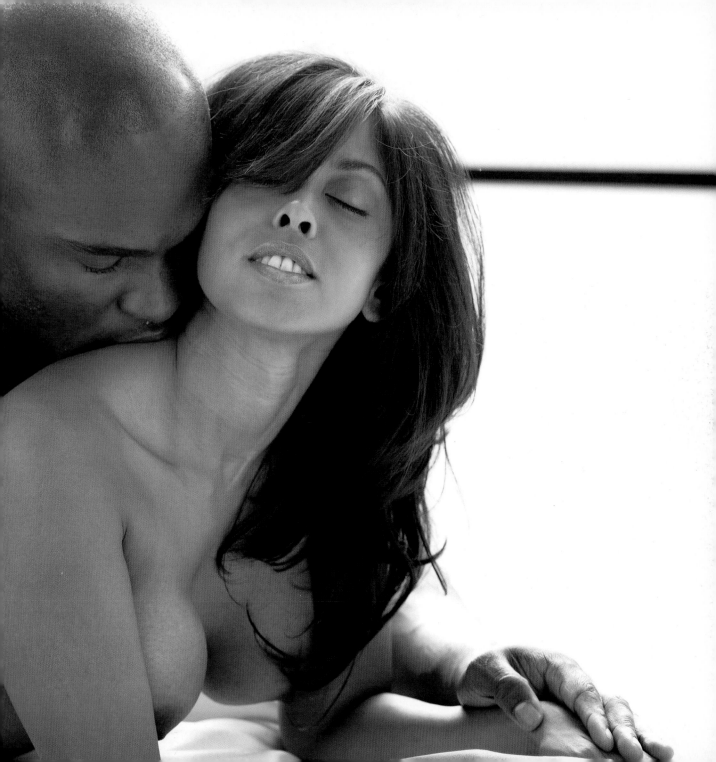

Hands-Free Clitoral Vibes

Sometimes, it's all about the rub. By which I mean, instead of taking a vibe and rubbing it against your body, some women would prefer to rub their clitoris against something with a lot of surface area. Others like the idea of a vibrator that you don't have to hold with your hands because they have more important things to do with their hands! Large round, cylindrical, or mostly round vibrators are perfect when you want to hold and squeeze something between your legs.

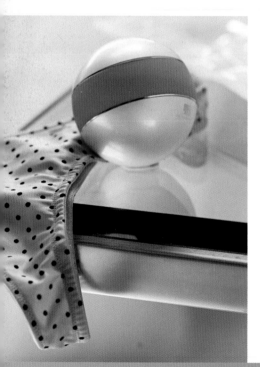

For example, the Tuyo by Big Teaze Toys ($65 to $75) is a round vibrator the size of a grapefruit with a diameter of about 3 inches (7.5 cm); it's made of stainless steel, phthalate-free plastics, and silicone. This sleek, modern toy challenges the notion that vibrators have to be phallic. The on/off switch is cleverly integrated into the design, so there are no protruding buttons; it has three speeds and five different vibration modes, which offer different kinds of pulsation. Women can use it in a number of ways by themselves or with a partner. Squeeze it between your legs, with the bottom half (where the vibration is concentrated) against your vulva. Lie on your stomach and slip it underneath you. Lie on your back, hold it between your legs, and have your partner straddle it so his balls rub against it as it vibrates against you.

Big Teaze also makes a toy called I Rub My Duckie ($25); it looks exactly like the wholesome rubber ducky you find in bathtubs across America, except it has a secret: It vibrates! It comes in two sizes and several different colors. On the surface, it may seem to be a funny gag gift for someone, but actually it's become quite a phenomenon, and plenty of women swear by this waterproof vibrator. If you're interested in finding one of the most innocuous-looking sex toys on the market, if you like to use a vibrator in the bath or shower, or if you're looking for moderate vibration and surface area in an adorable package, the I Rub My Duckie may be right up your alley.

The Cone Stands Alone

The Cone ($130) is a vibrator unlike any other. When you first see it, it looks strange. Yes, it's cone-shaped, as its name suggests, but it's a short, wide cone the size of a cantaloupe. It's made of silicone, runs on three C batteries, and is designed for hands-free pleasure. There are two buttons on one side of the base of the Cone, which offer sixteen different options to change the speed, type, and intensity of vibration. Because it has a flat bottom, it can sit on a level surface and will stay put. It has endless possibilities when it comes to self-pleasure. You can hold it between your legs and feel it vibrate against your vulva.

You can sit on it, with the pointed tip just inside your vagina or anus. You can lie on your stomach with it just underneath you. You can also use the Cone for partnered sex. Begin on all fours in Doggie-Style position with the Cone just underneath you, then move down until your vulva is resting against it; as your partner thrusts into you, he will push your body against the toy. In Spooning position, he can penetrate your anus while you hold the Cone between your legs with the pointed end inside your vagina. If he enjoys anal stimulation, he can sit on the Cone, then you can sit in his lap facing him in Yab-Yum position or facing away from him in Sitting Reverse Cowgirl. If you run out of ideas for using it, don't worry: it comes with a series of illustrations depicting women and men enjoying the Cone in all sorts of ways!

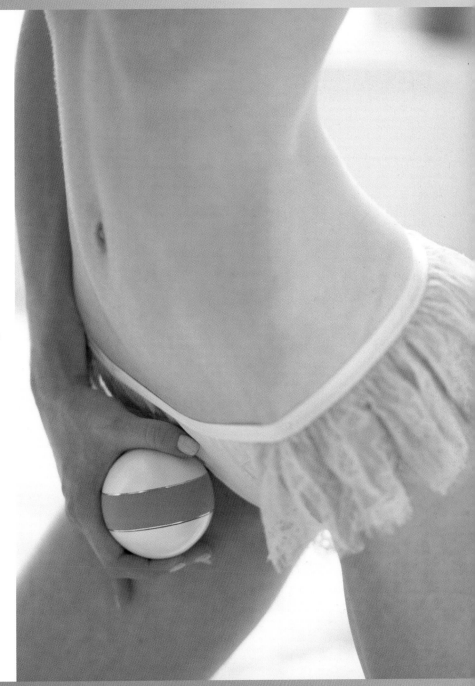

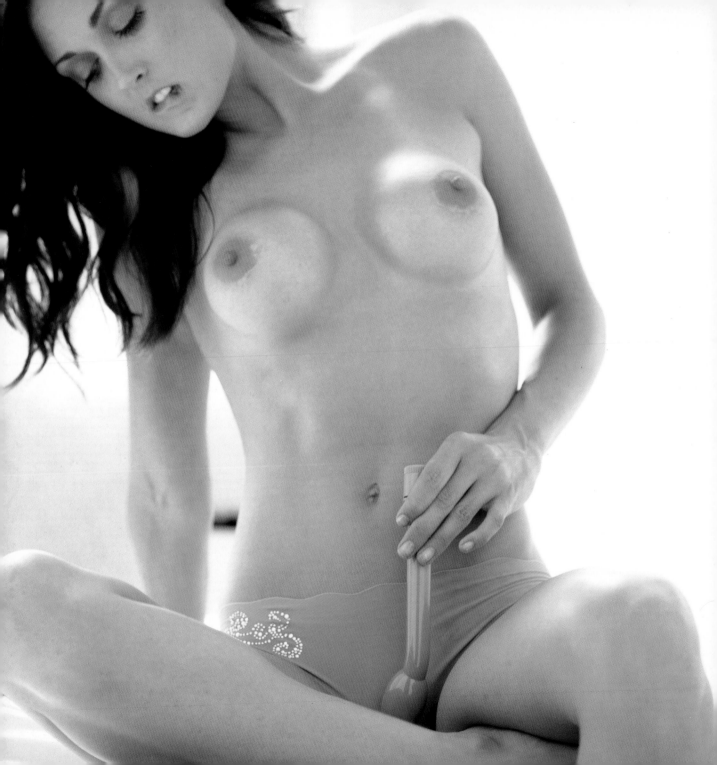

CHAPTER 9

WORK YOUR WAY IN WITH INSERTABLE VIBRATORS

Insertable vibrators are designed especially for penetration. They range in length (they can be as short as 4 inches [10 cm], but most tend to be about 7 to 8 inches [18 to 20 cm]) and girth and come in a variety of materials, textures, and styles. They are either battery-powered or rechargeable. Most are phallic-shaped, but not all of them are designed to look like penises. If you like penetration while you masturbate or are looking for a penetration toy that you can use with your partner, here are some of the most popular types of insertable vibrators.

Slimline Style: The Workhorse of Vibrators

The slimline is one of the classic, most recognizable styles of vibrator; it's one of the most abundant on the market and tends to be fairly inexpensive, making it good for beginners and people looking for an economical choice (about $15 to $25). Smooth and phallic, it looks like an oversized and elongated lipstick top and is about 7 to 8 inches (18 to 20 cm) long. You turn the cap on the base of the toy to turn it on and adjust the speed, and unscrew the cap to replace the batteries. Slimline vibrators are usually made of hard plastic or hard plastic covered in soft PVC and usually come in solid colors with the occasional animal or floral print; even those covered in soft PVC have a solid core, so these tend to be either rock hard or extremely firm. Either way, these toys are straight up and down and not flexible, and that can be a turn-off to some women who are looking for something curved or more flexible; some women find them uncomfortable for penetration because they're just too firm (read the end of this chapter for an alternative use for them).

Some of the less expensive vibes in this category are made of soft PVC or rubber, resemble a circumcised penis, and are softer and more flexible than the hard plastic slimline. They have a similar control mechanism as the slimline style: You turn the cap to control the speed. Many elements of the slimline put it comfortably in the middle of several spectrums: It's not the quietest, nor the loudest, of vibrators, but somewhere in between, and it delivers a medium intensity of vibration. Because the slimline does not have a flared base, you should only use it vaginally—never use it for anal penetration. The slimline does not promise high-tech features, a stunning design and aesthetic, or something unique; however, it's a solid workhorse of a vibrator, and personally, I always have one handy in my toy box!

Silicone Phallic Vibes: High Quality and Durable

If you like the shape of the slimline, but want a vibrator made of higher quality material with different textures and designs, then consider a silicone phallic vibe. Many of these vibrators are battery-operated, and some are rechargeable. German-based company Fun Factory makes the best line of silicone insertable vibrators—including favorites like Intensity ($160), Patchy Paul G2 ($70), and Gigolo ($70)—that are about 7 inches (18 cm) long and vary in width. Because they're silicone, they are durable, easy to clean, and warm to body temperature; plus, silicone conducts vibration well, making it an ideal material for vibrators. A few Fun Factory vibes vaguely resemble penises, but most feature a phallic shape with different

ripples, bumps, and textures on them; some are designed to look like sea creatures or signs of the Zodiac. If you like the design of the Fun Factory vibes but find them too big, the company also makes "mini" versions of its phallic vibes ($60 to $65), which are about 4 inches (10 cm) long. Like the slimline, these toys don't have a flared base, so they're best for vaginal penetration only.

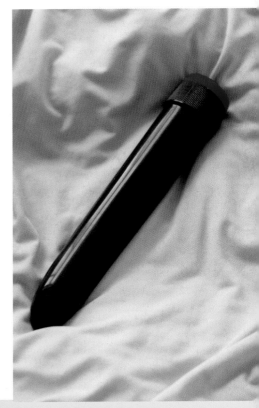

Slimline Vibe

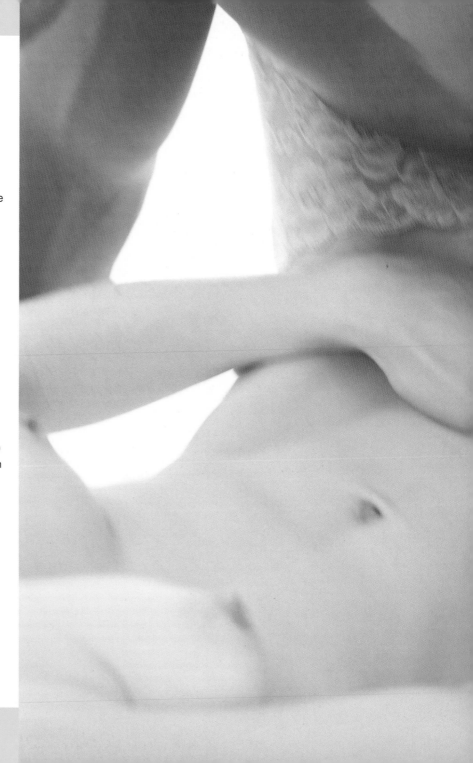

Perfect Pairing: Fun Factory Phantasy + Missionary Position

This is a great activity when you want to try out any new insertable vibrator or when she's ready for another round of penetration but your penis is done for the night. In Missionary position, the woman lies on her back and her partner sits up between her legs. Coat the Phantasy ($160) in her favorite lube, turn it on to the lowest setting, then tease her labia and vaginal opening with the tip of it. Take advantage of all the access you have to her body in this position: Kiss her, play with her hair, rub her nipples between your fingers, and stroke her inner thighs. Continue to tease her with the dildo just at her opening until she can't stand it anymore and she has to beg you to penetrate her. When she does, slide it inside only an inch (2.5 cm) to continue to build her anticipation. With your other hand, guide her hand down between her legs and ask her to touch herself—the combination of penetration and clitoral stimulation will feel amazing. Slide the vibrator in deeper and turn up the speed as you begin to establish a rhythm. In. Out. In. Out. Try out the different vibration modes and see which one she likes best.

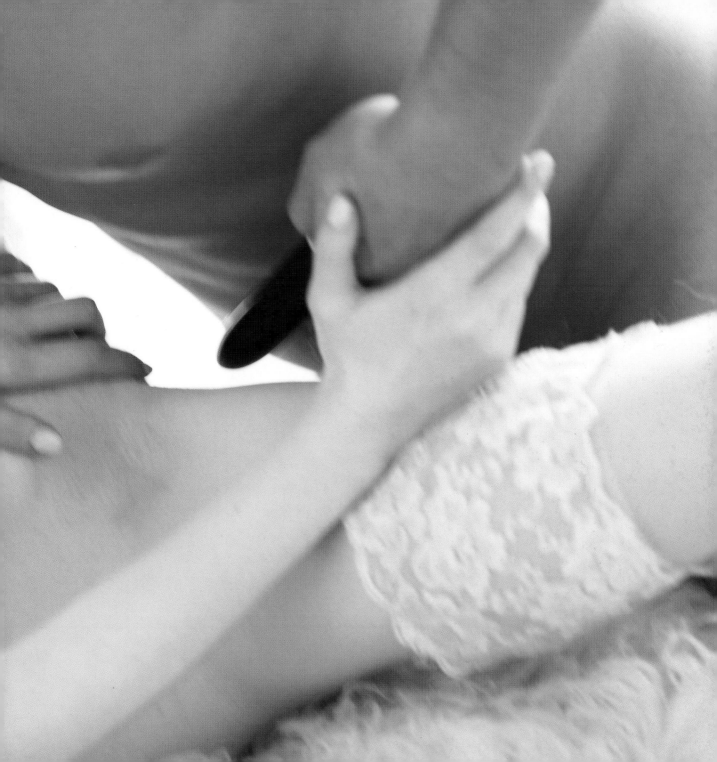

G-Spotters: Curved Heads Make the Vibe

Some insertable vibrators are designed specifically for G-spot stimulation, and you can tell because they have distinctively curved heads (as opposed to the straight style of slimline or phallic), and some have balls on the end of them; the curve is meant to aim directly for that sensitive spot on the front wall of the vagina. Most vibrators in this style are made of hard plastic, softer PVC, TPR, or silicone. The firmness of a G-spotter vibrator is part of what makes it work, because the G-spot responds well to hard toys and deliberate pressure during penetration. If you want something firm, smooth, and slim for penetration, try the Orchid G from Babeland ($22) or the Satin G by California Exotic Novelties ($15), which are both made of hard plastic and produce a moderate amount of vibration. Babeland's Nubby G ($25), made of pliable thermoplastic rubber, is shaped like a hooked finger. Halfway down the toy is a wider ring with textured nubs on it; when you slide it inside you, the nubs stimulate your clitoris in the front and the outside of your anus in the back. So if you're looking for a G-spot vibe that's flexible and provides additional external stimulation, it's a good bet. The staff of one of the first women-run sex shops, Good Vibrations, designed their own line of vibrators, and two of them are all about the G-spot. The G Twist ($65) is a silicone curved vibe that has a ridged texture all along its shaft and one exaggerated ridge near the bottom to stimulate the clitoris when it's inside you. The G Swirl ($65) is also silicone and has a shape similar to the Nubby G without the nubs on the wider ring portion; because of the wide ring, both these toys can be used vaginally and anally.

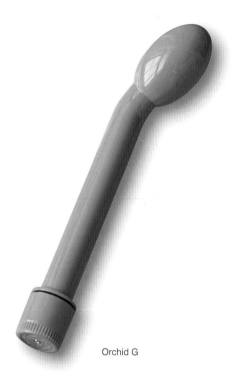

Orchid G

How to Find the G-Spot

The urethra is surrounded by the urethral sponge (also known as the G-spot), which is made of spongy erectile tissue that contains paraurethral glands and ducts. You can feel the G-spot through the front wall of the vagina, about 1 to 2 inches (2.5 to 5 cm) inside the vaginal opening. Like the clitoris, the G-spot is not just an isolated spot of sensitivity, but part of a network of nerves, muscles, and tissue. When a woman is turned on, the glands within the urethral sponge fill with fluid, causing the sponge to swell; as it becomes more pronounced, it's easier to find and more sensitive to stimulation. The more turned on a woman is, the easier it will be to find her G-spot. So, before you go hunting for it and especially before you start stimulating it, make sure you warm her up.

To find the G-spot, it's best to start with your fingers, because our sense of touch is keen and connected right back to the brain. Make sure your fingernails are clean, short, and well filed before you begin any penetration with them. If you're not sure about your nails, slip on a latex or nonlatex glove to transform your fingers into smooth tools. Slide a finger inside 1 to 1½ inches (2.5 to 4 cm) and aim toward the front wall of the vagina. If you stroke the area, you should be able to locate the G-spot. Compared to the smoother tissue of the inside of the vagina, the G-spot will have a different texture: It will feel wrinkled or ridged. One of the best techniques to use with your fingers is a "come here" motion. With your fingers inside your partner and against the front wall of the vagina, move your fingers toward you and down slightly as if you're saying "come here." It's almost like you are trying to pull the spot out of her. Be sure to warm her up with your fingers before using a toy.

Once you've found her spot and she's turned on, lube up the G-spot vibrator and slide it inside her. Remember, the G-spot is only an inch or two (2.5 to 5 cm) inside, so you don't have to go all the way in to reach it. You want to aim the curved head of the vibrator at her G-spot. Some women like to have the toy pressed against the G-spot with only a little bit of movement while the vibration does most of the stimulation. Others like an in-and-out motion and can feel the head of the vibrator hit the G-spot as the toy slides in, then out again.

Alternate Uses: They're Not Just Insertable!

Most people assume that when they see a phallic-shaped vibrator that it's meant for penetration. While all the vibrators and styles covered in this chapter are insertable—and many are designed specifically for penetration and G-spot stimulation—they all have another function as well: You can use any of them as clitoral vibrators. That's right! Don't be fooled by the label "insertable"; many of these vibrators work just as well for clitoral stimulation. In fact, because most of them are about 7 inches (18 cm) long and 1¼ to 2 inches (3 to 5 cm) in diameter, they have plenty of surface area to cover the clitoris and surrounding parts of the vulva. Simply hold the vibrator parallel to your torso and press the bottom half of it against your clitoris. How's that for a versatile toy?!

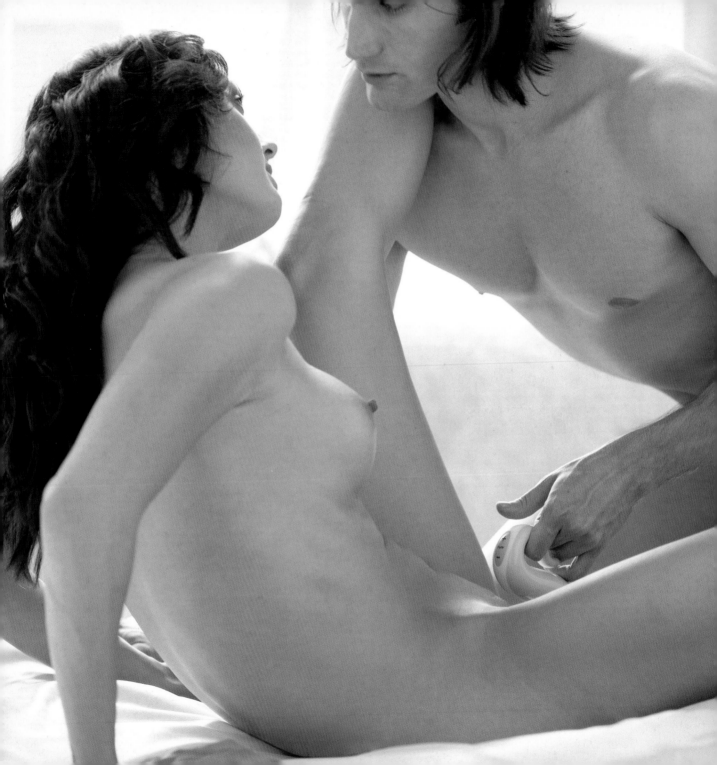

CHAPTER 10

TWICE AS NICE:

Dual-Action Vibrators

For many women, the key to intense pleasure and orgasm is the perfect combination of penetration and clitoral stimulation delivered at the same time. Makers of dual-action vibrators know this and have created toys meant to excite all of her most sensitive spots simultaneously. Are you a woman who likes to have your cake and eat it, too? If you ultimately want the best of both worlds when it comes to toys that vibrate, then a dual-action vibrator is the right choice for you.

Rabbit Style Hits Two Spots

The basic concept behind the rabbit-style dual-action vibrator is to combine an insertable vibrator with a clitoral vibrator into one toy and give each vibrating part separate controls. I call this kind of toy "rabbit style" because the Rabbit Pearl ($80 to $90) is the most well-known toy in this category, made famous by Samantha in *Sex and the City*. The designs of these toys are pretty universal: a phallic-shaped shaft with a clitoral attachment that often resembles a cute little animal.

There are more than a hundred rabbit-style vibrators on the market from dozens of different manufacturers, and they all have subtle design differences as well as varied features. The control and battery unit is either at the base of the shaft or it's a separate unit attached by a wire; some people like the convenience of having everything in one unit, whereas others find it easier to adjust the controls when they are separate from the vibrator. Rabbit-style vibrators can be made of rubber, jelly rubber, PVC, elastomer, TPR, or silicone. The silicone dual-action vibrators are the most resilient and easiest to clean. The insertable part of the vibrator can have various features. In addition to vibrating, some shafts are bendable, so you can change not only the speed of the vibration but also the angle of its orbit. Some shafts have a ring of beads at the bottom that rotate; the ring is meant to stimulate the vaginal opening, which is the most sensitive part of the vagina.

The clitoral attachment also varies from toy to toy. You can choose an animal, which will deliver a light fluttering motion against your clitoris, usually with its ears, paws, or antennae. Or, if you like more pressure against your clit, pick a toy with a more solid (usually nonanimal) attachment—think more like an oval bullet—so you have something firmer to rub against. Keep in mind that depending on the design, the clitoral attachment may sit away from the clitoris or may not hug your clitoris close enough once the toy is inside you; simply take your hand and hold it against you.

Vibratex, which manufacturers its toys in Japan, is considered the leader in dual-action vibes, and you'll find several of their styles on my list of Top Picks for Rabbit-Style Vibes.

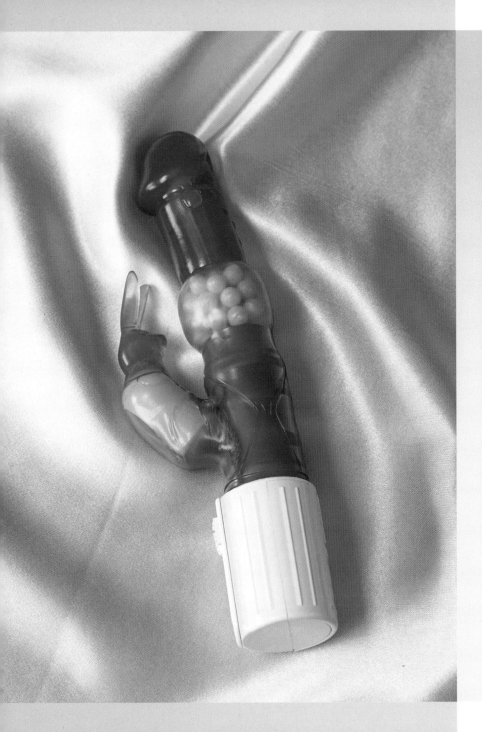

Tristan's Top Picks for Rabbit-Style Vibes

If You Want . . .

A gentle fluttering motion on your clit: Butterfly by Vibratex ($95)

A rotating ring of beads in the shaft: Rabbit Habit by Vibratex ($80 to $90)

Something nice and big: Twice as Titan by Vibratex ($150)

Inexpensive but high quality: Thumbelina by Vibratex ($40 to $50)

Triple action (vaginal, clitoral, and anal): Dr. Ava's Trigasm by Doc Johnson ($100 to $140)

A textured shaft with a curve for G-spot stimulation: Paul & Paulina by Fun Factory ($75 to $80)

Rotating shaft without the clit attachment: Beehive at Early to Bed ($40)

Smooth, streamlined, and to the point: Wilma at Early to Bed ($28)

Why Does My Vibrator Have a Face on It?

The dual-action vibrator design originated in Japan, where it happens to be illegal to make anatomically correct sex toys. So, in order to skirt the law and still make a phallic-shaped toy, designers transformed what looks like the ridge of a circumcised penis head into a person's head with a face on the front and a thick head of hair on top. Then, they made the clitoral attachments into cute little animals. Although companies in different parts of the world have copied the design, Japan still has a reputation for making some of the best-quality vibrators; if your vibrator has a face on it, chances are it's from Japan.

Curved for Double Action

It used to be that rabbit-style vibes were the only ones that delivered simultaneous penetration and clitoral stimulation, but there is a new group of multitaskers on the market that have joined the party. These are very different in shape from the phallic rabbit style; they tend to be curvy U and S shapes. The first is the Rock Chick ($60 to $70), a silicone U-shaped, battery-powered vibrator made by British company Rocks Off Ltd. The smooth part of the Rock Chick goes inside your vagina, and its exaggerated curve targets the sensitive G-spot, while the ridged end hugs your clitoris and vulva. Rather than using the toy like a traditional dildo with a straight in-and-out motion, you make a much shallower rocking motion with the Rock Chick. As you do, the toy stimulates the G-spot and the clitoris at the same time.

Vibratex makes a toy with a similar design called the Snuggle Puss ($35 to $45), although its surface is more textured with bumps throughout, and it's designed so you can wear it for hands-free fun. Speaking of a good time, Fun Factory makes a toy called Delight ($130), a silicone and plastic S-shaped, recharge-able vibrator with an elegant design and controls built into it that light up. Hold on to the ergonomic curvy handle, slide the hooked silicone end inside your vagina for great G-spot stimulation, and the middle of the S vibrates against your clitoris.

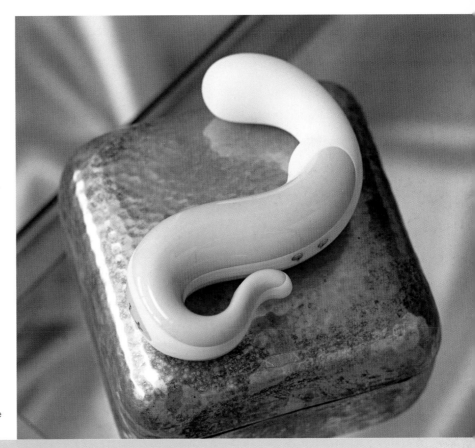

Delight Vibe

Perfect Pairing: Delight Vibe + Inverted Spider Position

To get into this position, she begins by lying on her back and he kneels between her legs. She raises her legs up and he pulls her ankles toward his shoulders. Then, she lifts her pelvis up and off the bed so that she's supporting her weight on her upper back and shoulders. If this is too uncomfortable for her, try using a Liberator Shape (see page 188) to achieve the right angle and get some support under her body. Once she's in position, lube the end of the Delight and tease her with it. Slide it inside her slowly, and once it's inside, have her adjust the vibration. With the easy-to-use handle, you can move the toy in and out of her, massaging the G-spot each time you do. The Inverted Spider position allows partners to face each other for optimal communication and eye contact. He has a perfect view of her entire body, which is at an ideal angle for G-spot stimulation, plus he can maneuver the vibrator easily because of its shape. She can also take a turn holding the toy, while he supports her body and enjoys the show. All the blood rushes to her head in this position, which may intensify sensations and orgasms for some women.

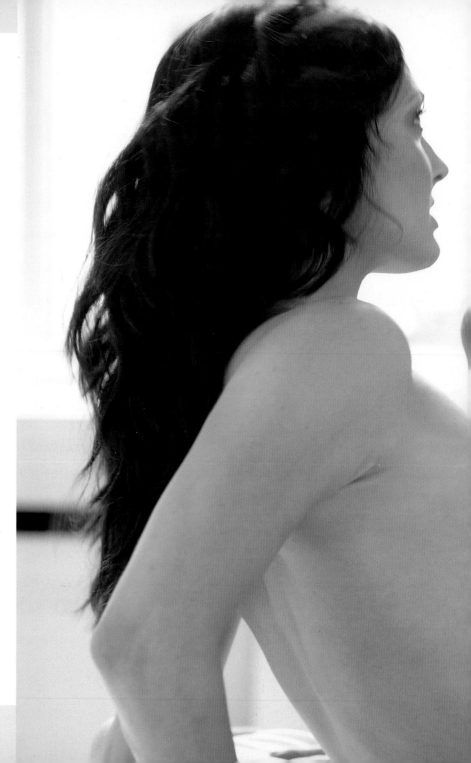

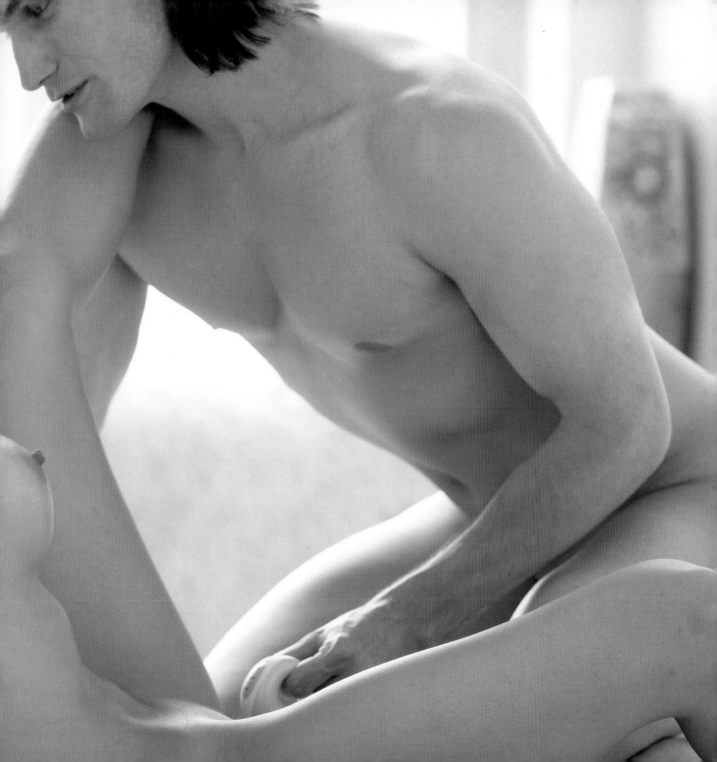

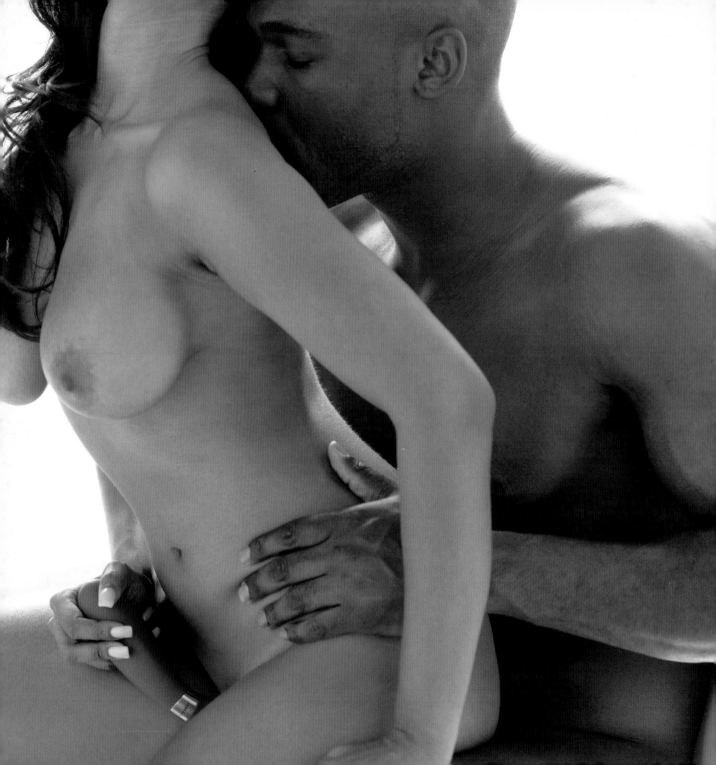

CHAPTER 11

HIGH-TECH AND LUXURY VIBRATORS:
Smart and Sassy

Whether it's how we communicate with each other, get our entertainment, or do our jobs, technology plays a big role in our lives. So it's only fitting that technology also plays a role in our sex lives. The makers of the vibrators in this chapter use technology in creative ways that put them on the cutting edge of sex toy design. These are the next generation of vibrators, and we're going to see more like them in the future. They do things other vibrators (or sex toys) cannot, making them "smarter" than typical vibrators. These toys are perfect for gadget lovers, high-tech geeks, and folks who want the latest, hottest new thing. As you might expect, their price tag usually reflects their high-tech qualities, but ultimately you're worth it!

Smart Vibrator: The SaSi

SaSi ($185) is the first vibrator of its kind, made by London-based company Je Joue and distributed exclusively in the United States by Babeland. It has a sleek design that hugs a woman's body, it's made of medical-grade silicone, and it's environmentally friendly because it's rechargeable. At first glance, SaSi looks like another high-end, top-quality, ergonomically designed clitoral vibrator. It is, but it's also more. Instead of simply having the surface of the toy vibrate against the body, a small ball underneath the soft silicone surface moves as it vibrates. It has five different vibration options, which combine vibration and movement to create a different sensation than your typical vibrator—it's more like a gentle, but deliberate, kneading sensation that also vibrates. Like to have your clit rubbed up one side of the hood and down the other? There's a mode for that. What about back and forth in a more concentrated space? There's a mode for that. It's this combination of movement and vibration that sets it apart from typical vibrators. Women who find the basic vibrator too intense, too much like a jackhammer, or not subtle enough to move against their body the way they like should definitely try the SaSi. If you love cunnilingus and wish a vibrator could better simulate the sensations of oral sex, SaSi is it. Here's the best part: It actually learns what you like. In Favorites mode, you choose from five different vibration modes. In Customize mode, it switches automatically from one vibration mode to the next. If you don't like one, you hit skip; if you love one, you hit another button; the SaSi remembers what you liked and will customize the modes it goes through the next time you use it.

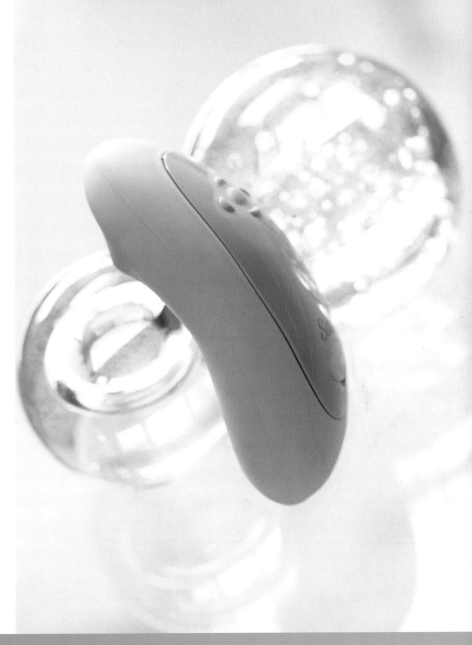

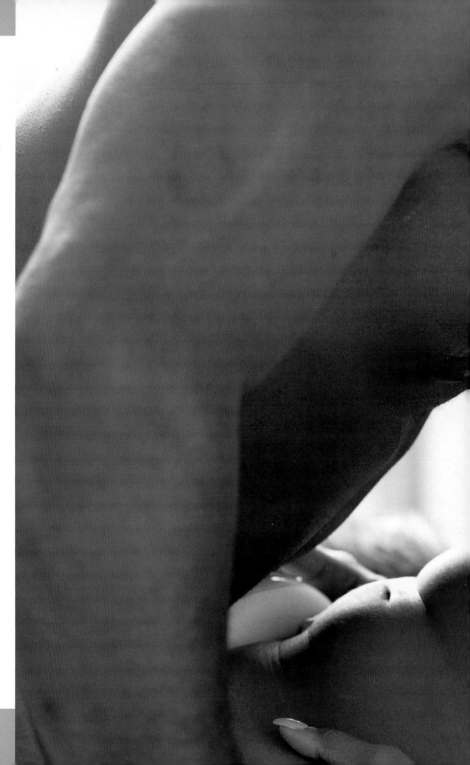

Perfect Pairing: SaSi + Upright Missionary Position

In Upright Missionary position, she lies on her back, he sits up on his knees and positions himself between her legs, and she bends her knees. In this position, he can caress and squeeze her breasts or even pinch her nipples if she likes it; both partners can easily reach and stimulate her clitoris with the SaSi vibrator. He has a good view of the action in this position, because he can watch his penis go in and out of her. She can look at him as he penetrates her and stroke his chest and nipples. This can be an alternative to Missionary if she wants his weight off of her; it's also good for partners of very different heights or weights. For a woman who wishes she could combine oral sex with intercourse, this is your recipe!

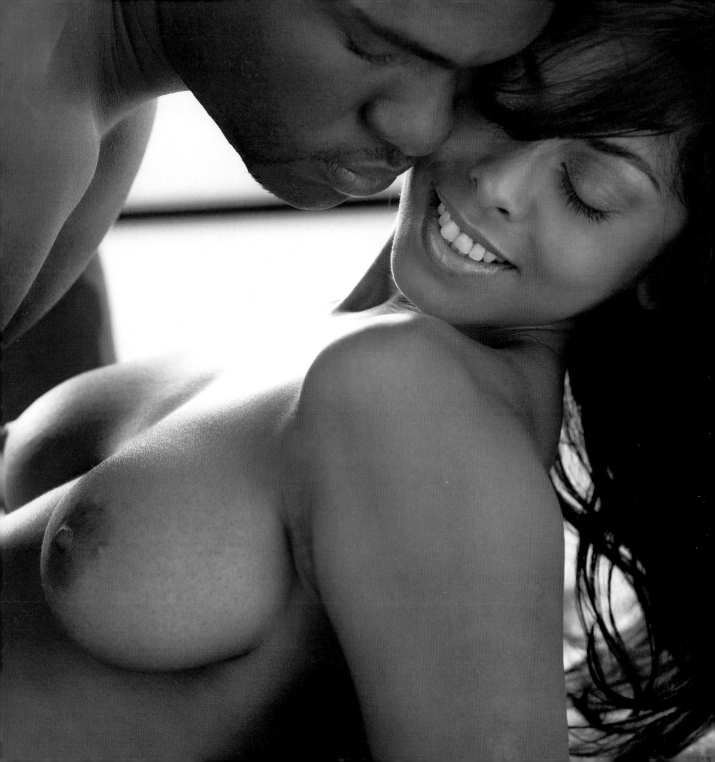

MP3- and Cell Phone-Compatible Vibes: Bring Your Gadgets into the Bedroom

Sex and music are natural companions: The right music can really get you in a good frame of mind, set a seductive mood, and enhance the erotic experience. OhMiBod was the first company to develop a vibrator that's compatible with MP3 players like iPods. You connect the OhMiBod vibrator ($70) to your iPod, and it pulses to the rhythm of the music. When the vibration is tuned to the beat of the music, it produces a very unique experience. For music lovers and those who can't live without their iPods, this toy is a must-have. Although it's designed for use with a portable MP3 player, you can actually hook it up to lots of different electronics, including laptops, stereos, portable CD players, microphones, and even electric guitars (bringing a whole new meaning to "intense jam session").

The original OhMiBod is a hard plastic, bullet-shaped vibrator that's 5½ inches (13.75 cm) long and made for clitoral stimulation or vaginal penetration. The company makes several other designs, including the Naughtibod ($70), which has a velvety texture and a rippled shape—a definite upgrade on the original.

The same company makes vibrators that work with your cell phone. The Boditalk ($70) and Boditalk Escort ($60) are activated when someone who's nearby calls your cell phone. The call triggers the vibration, which continues for as long as you talk—perfect for those folks who like to have phone sex, want to do something naughty in public, and love gadgets.

Wireless Vibrators Offer Remote-Controlled Action

For couples who like to play games, there are remote-controlled vibrators. Imagine if you tucked an egg vibrator discreetly in your panties, held it between your legs so it was right up against your clitoris, or slid it inside your vagina. Now think about what it would be like if you couldn't control the vibrator, but your partner held the controls and you were at his mercy! That's right, he can turn it (and you) on and off, and change the speed and vibration mode whenever he wants. Your job: Take as much as he can dish out.

Remote-controlled vibrators are fun to play with at home, where your partner can tease you, taunt you, and bring you to the edge of orgasm with the touch of a button. If you like to be teased or told you can't come just yet, this vibrator is for you. These vibes are also great for couples who want to go out in public with a secret. Imagine sitting down at a nice restaurant, going to the theater, or hanging out at a party while one of you has a vibrator under her clothes and the other one has his finger on the button! It's a great way to make dinner with the neighbors more interesting, bring some spice to the movie theater, or add a sexy layer to a party that only the two of you know about.

OhMiBod and Naughtybod

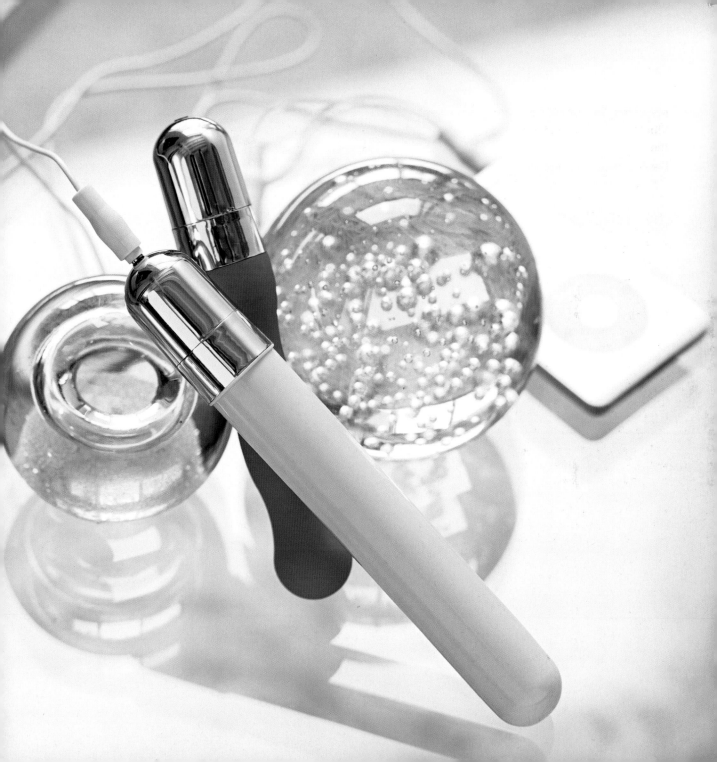

Luxury Vibrators Combine Superior Quality and Technology, Plus Marketing

What makes a vibrator luxurious? Superior design, top-quality materials, advanced technology, and a hefty price tag all contribute to luxury vibes being in a class by themselves. Let's face it, it's also about marketing. Just like it's sometimes hard to distinguish a pair of $30 jeans from a pair of $200 jeans, part of it is branding and marketing—you're paying for the name. Two of the top luxury toy companies are Lelo and Jimmyjane.

Lelo is a Swedish company that makes vibrators and other toys that are gorgeously designed and packaged. Their vibrators are very well made and especially quiet (I recommended their compact ergonomic clitoral vibrator Nea in chapter 6). Two of their most popular toys are the insertable vibes Liv and Gigi. Both are made of medical-grade silicone and hard plastic, and they are rechargeable; they stay charged for about an hour.

The Liv ($109) is 6½ inches (16.25 cm) long (with 4½ inches [11.25 cm] making up the insertable portion) and has a very subtle curve. If you've found that insertable vibrators are too big or G-spot vibes with an exaggerated curve aren't comfortable for you, the Liv may be a perfect fit. It also has pretty strong vibration and works just as well as an external clitoral vibrator. The Gigi ($109) is similar in design but thicker and has a firm raised end to target the G-spot. Both toys have five different vibration modes: a constant vibration, three pulsing vibrations (slow, medium, and fast intervals), and "before and after" mode, where the vibration builds to a strong surge, then backs off, then builds again, etc. You can control both the mode *and* the speed, offering many possibilities.

The Form 6 ($185) by high-end retailer Jimmyjane is also silicone with metal and plastic trim; it's waterproof and rechargeable (it holds a charge for up to 2 hours).

The Form 6 is curved at both ends with three buttons in the middle, designed so that you can use either end of the vibrator for penetration or for external clitoral stimulation. It has a body-conscious ergonomic design, and works better as an external vibrator than an insertable one. However, one of the cool features of the Form 6 is that if you insert the smaller end inside the vagina, the outer portion sits right against the vulva and clitoris, making it a dual-action insertable vibrator. It has six vibration modes: One is a constant, even vibration; three are wavelike, where the vibration builds up, then down; and two are pulsing, with pulses at different speeds. Each end has a separate motor, so in each mode, the small end and larger end vibrate in slightly different ways.

Form 6

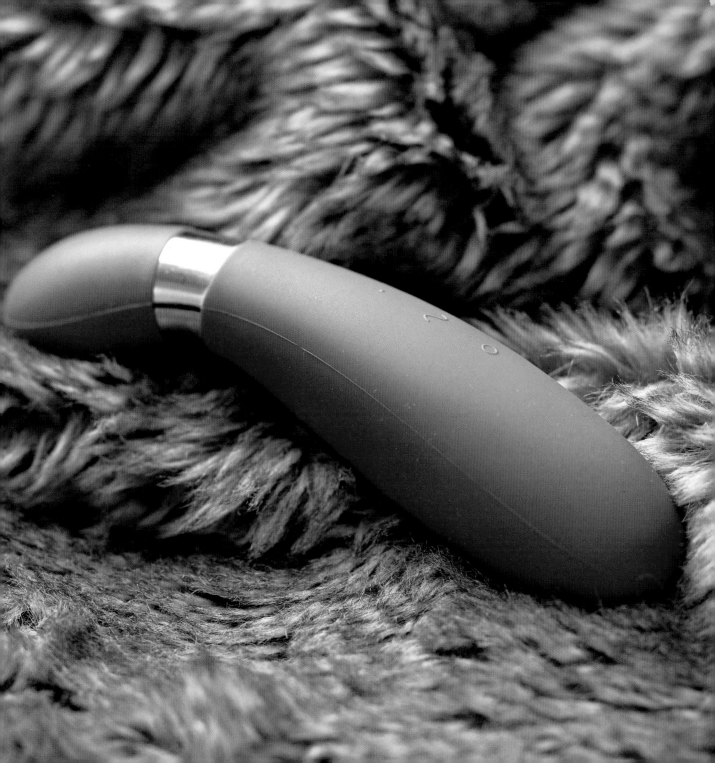

Web-Enabled Vibrators Take Cybersex to a New Level

Whether you're in a long-distance relationship or just like to have fun with your computer, the Internet is a place where we often connect with our partners through instant messages, email, chatting, and Web cams. People already have cybersex online, so why not have cybersex while you play with a Web-enabled vibrator? Web-enabled vibrators are vibrators that can be connected to one computer and controlled by someone online from his or her computer. HighJoy.com and Doc Johnson teamed up to create an egg vibrator, a rabbit vibe, and a penis sleeve that are Internet-ready ($60, $85, $70). For them to work, you must subscribe to HighJoy's website, where your encounters have to take place. Basically, an image of the toy's control appears on the screen, you move the controls with your mouse, and the toy at the other end responds.

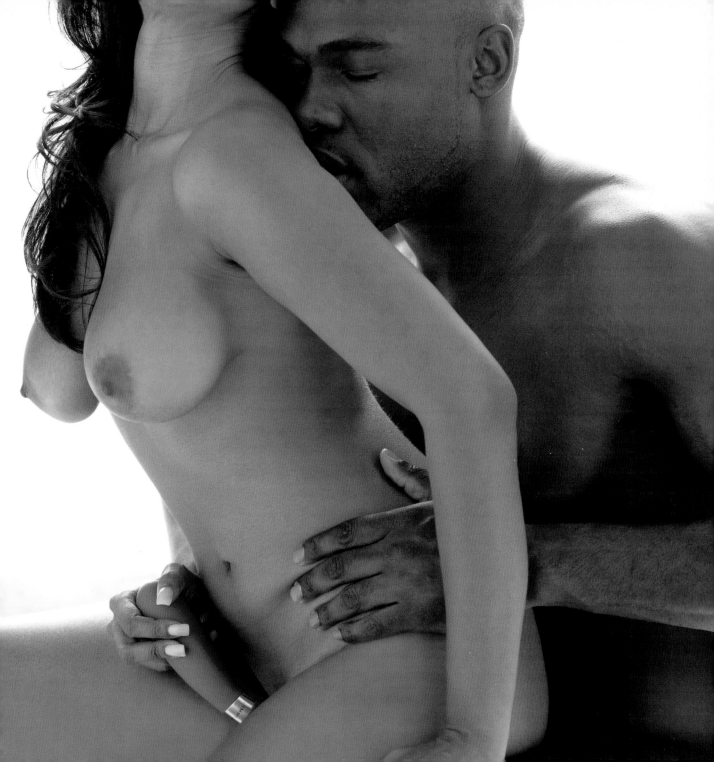

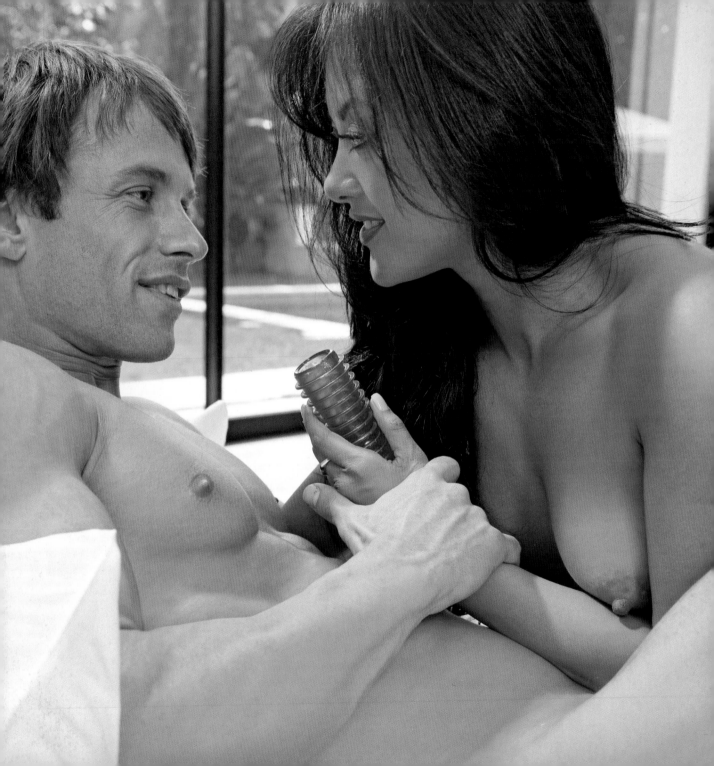

CHAPTER 12

PLEASURE FOR HIM:

Penis Sleeves and Pumps

Penis sleeves and pumps are among the most popular masturbation toys for men. Just like for women, masturbation is an important part of a man's sex life. It's a chance for him to connect with his body, explore his sexual desires and fantasies, try new things, and get better acquainted with his likes and dislikes. Masturbation is not just for single men or men who are away from their partners! Regardless of your sexual activity, all men should take time out of their busy lives to masturbate, and penis sleeves and pumps are a great way to experience new sensations or spice up your self-pleasure routine. If you want to learn to prolong intercourse, using a penis sleeve is a great way to practice how to control and delay ejaculation. Some men use penis pumps not just for masturbation, but to help them achieve an erection or get a stronger one.

Penis Sleeves Give Him a Helping Hand

Sleeves are made of jelly rubber, PVC, elastomer, thermal plastics (with trademarked names like CyberSkin and Real Feel Super Skin), or silicone and come in a variety of styles. Most sleeves have some kind of texture on the inside, both to stimulate sensitive parts of the penis and to simulate intercourse. Some sleeves have a simple, tubular design with a hole at both ends, while others have openings designed to look like a mouth, a vagina, or an anus. Some sleeves are molded from the genitals of adult film stars.

Sleeves come in one size and tend to be quite stretchy to accommodate many different-sized penises. If you're looking for an especially snug fit, some companies make "extra tight" versions. All sleeves feature a textured interior with nubs, bumps, ridges, tendrils, or nodules. Some are contoured to feel like the walls of a vagina. Some have ridges or tight rings at the opening to simulate the opening of a vagina or an anus. Some penis sleeves can be inexpensive, but buyer beware: Those made of inferior materials and construction can tear easily, rendering the toy useless. Do your research, read toy reviews on websites, and ask a salesperson for a recommendation.

Before using a sleeve, put it into a bowl of very warm or hot water. This will warm the toy and make it feel more like skin. Shake the excess water out, then pour your favorite lube into the opening and coat your penis with lube as well. (Remember never to use silicone lubes with silicone or thermal plastic sleeves.) Lube is an important component for sleeves to work well. The idea is straightforward: You slide your penis into the sleeve, and the material grips it snuggly. As you move the sleeve up and down, the texture and tightness of the sleeve stimulates the penis, a sensation similar to having intercourse. You can also hold the sleeve still and move in and out of the sleeve; this technique works best with a sleeve like the Fleshlight, which is housed in a hard case (see page 126 for more

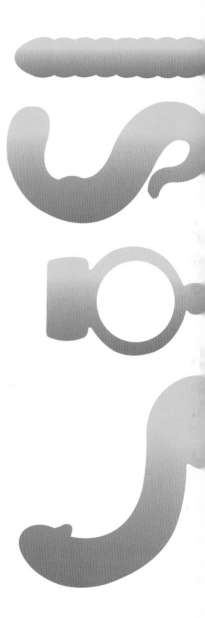

information on the Fleshlight). You can also wedge a sleeve between the mattress and box spring of your bed for hands-free thrusting; this works best if the height of your bed allows you to stand or kneel comfortably when you do it. Some sleeves have vibrators attached to them for extra stimulation; you can also use any vibrator at the end of a sleeve.

Although they are more difficult to find, there are also penis sleeves that are designed for a man to slip over his penis and wear during intercourse. The sleeve adds both length and girth to his penis, has a texture to stimulate his partner's vagina, and often vibrates. One of the best in this category is the Vibrating O Sleeve available at Babeland.

To maintain a sleeve's texture and make it last, it's important to clean and dry the sleeve thoroughly right after you use it. Some sleeves can be cleaned with mild soap and water or a sex toy cleaner, while others can only be cleaned with water. Follow instructions on the package.

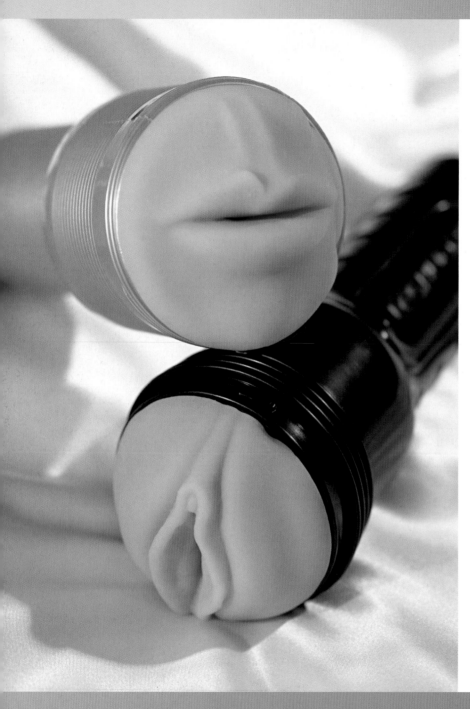

The Fleshlight: Rave Reviews All Around

The Fleshlight ($60) is the top penis sleeve on the market, a unique product that garners rave reviews from men everywhere. A guy once told me that using a Fleshlight was better than sex with a condom, it felt that great! Unlike other sleeves, this sleeve sits in a plastic casing (which looks like a giant flashlight, hence the name). Because it's in a case, it creates an amazing suction sensation. Plus, you can turn the cap on the end to increase or decrease the amount of suction. You can also remove the cap altogether and stick a small vibrator in the hole on the end to vibrate against the head of the penis. It's made of a patented phthalate-free plastic called Real Feel Super Skin that has an extremely realistic fleshlike texture.

You can remove the sleeve itself for cleaning, and the manufacturer recommends that you only clean it with warm water (no soap), shake out the excess water, and let it dry. After it dries, you must dust it with cornstarch—only cornstarch, never baby powder or talc. This helps it maintain its unique texture. If you don't dust it, it will become extremely sticky and tacky and impossible to use.

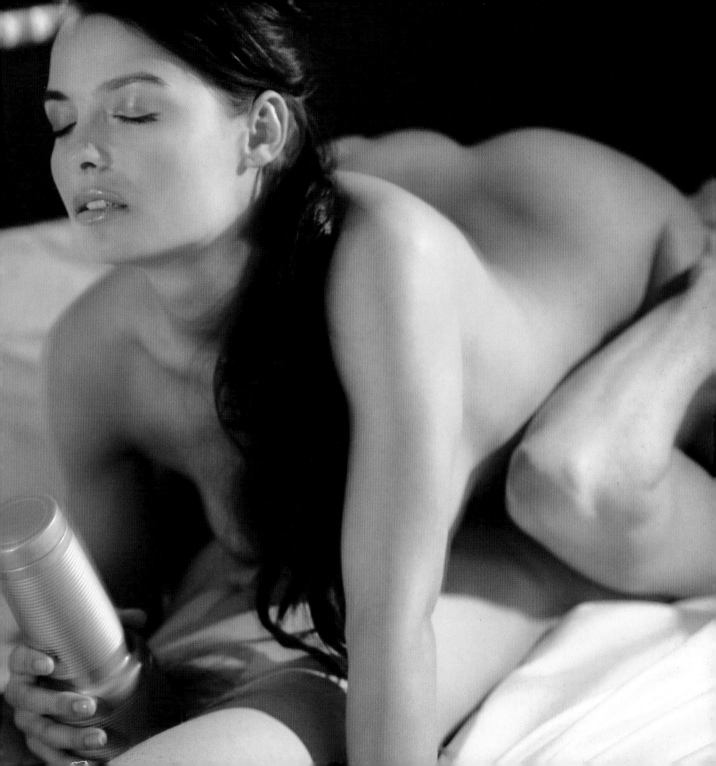

Penis Pumps Won't Change His Size but *Will* Make Him Hard

Penis pumps have a cylinder and an air pump; once you create a vacuum seal, you force air out of the cylinder with the pump. That draws blood into the penis, sparking the engorgement process and giving a man an erection. Men use penis pumps for a variety of reasons: they enjoy the suction sensation; to help them get an erection; to help them get a stronger erection; or to get an erection that lasts longer. Regardless of some marketing claims, penis pumps cannot and will not make your penis bigger. Some men do say that after long-term use, the shaft of the penis is better defined (just as other muscles in the body become more well defined after working out). If you have diabetes, circulatory problems, certain types of erectile dysfunction, cancer, or another serious medical condition, consult a physician before using a penis pump.

There are essentially two different kinds of pumps, which I call the basic pump ($20 to $50) and the advanced pump ($60 to $140); the cylinders in either kind are made of plastic or thin acrylic. A basic pump is a cylinder connected to a tube with a soft oval-shaped hand-squeeze pump on the end. Basic pumps tend to be less expensive than advanced pumps, and they're a good place to start if you've never bought a pump before and are not sure whether you'll like it. These pumps usually have a hole on top or the side that you have to cover while you pump and uncover to release the pressure once you have an erection. An advanced pump has a cylinder connected to tubing that's connected to a pistol-grip pump; the pump has a pressure gauge on it and a quick release tab. Some say these are safer because you can see how much you are pumping on the gauge; you can also note the exact number on the gauge to remember for next time. The quick release tab means it is more convenient because you don't have to hold your finger or hand over a hole, since your hand can slip in the process.

Some penis pumps have vibrators attached to them for extra stimulation during the pumping process. Some have attachments you can put on the opening that are made of a softer material (such as jelly rubber, silicone, or thermal plastic); the soft attachment sits around the base of your penis and makes it more comfortable and pleasurable for some, kind of like combining a penis sleeve and a pump into one toy.

To use a penis pump, rub lube around the flared opening of the cylinder and on the base of your penis; the idea is to create a vacuum seal. If you're having

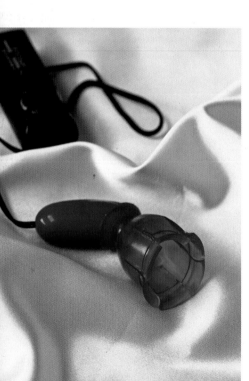

The Hugger

trouble creating a tight seal, you may need more lube or you may need to trim or shave your pubic hair. Put the cylinder over your penis. If there is a hole in the top or on one side, cover it with your finger or hand. With the hand pump, give it one or two pumps and see how it feels. If you have extra skin or the skin of your scrotal sac is loose, it can get sucked into the cylinder, which some people like. If you want to avoid that, hold your sac away from the cylinder as you pump. Go slowly and never pump to the point that it hurts. You should also never pump for more than 15 minutes. Once you have an erection, stop pumping and leave the cylinder on for a few minutes; this will continue the engorgement process. Release the air from the cylinder by removing your hand from the hole or using a quick release valve, if the pump has one.

Pumping while in the shower or bath is fun, because the genital tissue is warm and can expand easier, but make sure you have a waterproof, bath-safe pump. You can also pump right after a hot shower or bath. Some men like to put on a cock ring after pumping to maintain the effects; you can read more about cock rings in the next chapter.

Vibrator for Him: The Hugger

The Hugger ($20) is a vibrator designed especially for penis stimulation. It's basically a bullet-shaped vibrator with a cup attachment that resembles an upside-down tulip. The cup hugs the head, and the petals vibrate against it, delivering vibration to the most sensitive part of the penis.

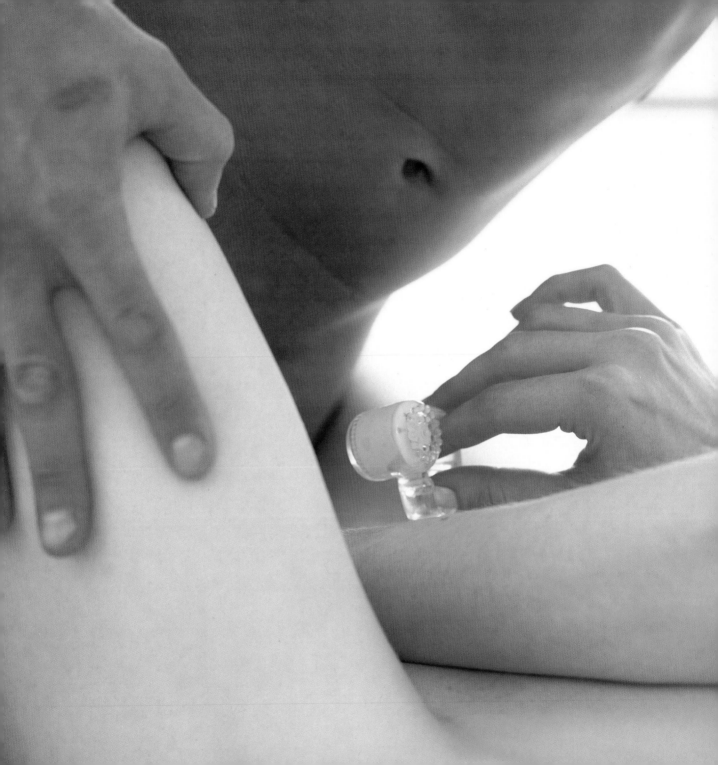

CHAPTER 13

ALL YOU EVER WANTED TO KNOW ABOUT COCK RINGS

A cock ring is a ring of material that a man wears around the base of his penis and scrotal sac; it stops blood from moving away from the penis to make orgasm more intense. Men use cock rings for many different reasons:

- To create the sensation that something is holding onto the penis and balls

- To help maintain a stronger, firmer erection

- To keep an erection for a longer period of time

- To make the penis more sensitive to all kinds of stimulation

- To prolong intercourse

- To delay ejaculation

Soft Nonadjustable Cock Rings: Inexpensive but Hard to Fit

The most basic of all cock rings are the smooth continuous O-rings that look like small bracelets ($6 to $30). They can be made of rubber, nitrile, or silicone and come in a variety of different diameters. They are inexpensive (silicone being the priciest in this category), are easy to find, and will get the job done. If you are trying a cock ring for the first time, not sure what it's all about, and don't want to spend a bunch of money, then a continuous ring is a good place to start. The biggest drawback of the basic cock ring is that it's one size and not very adjustable. Some men find that it becomes uncomfortable after a while because it's not the perfect size and there's no way to change it but to take it off. The rubber and silicone have some give to them. Silicone rings are better quality, last longer, and are easy to clean. Nitrile rings are slightly more flexible, and nitrile is a safe, latex-free alternative for those men or their partners who are sensitive or allergic to latex.

Given this drawback, the most important element of a nonadjustable cock ring is the fit. It's best to measure yourself while hard to determine which size ring will work for you. Take a soft tape measure (or a string that you can later put against a regular ruler) and measure the distance around the cock and balls (at the base, behind the scrotum). Divide this number by 3.1. For example, if you measure 4.5 inches (11.25 cm), then you want a cock ring with a 1½-inch (3.75-cm) diameter. If you come up with an odd number, always get the bigger size. Don't try to eyeball this one; ask the store clerk, or if you're shopping online, reputable websites will note the diameter of the ring in the product description.

Jelly rubber rings usually have the most stretch to them. In general, the stretchier the ring, the easier it is to put on and fit properly. Some of these types of cock rings have ridges or bumps on one side.

These rings are designed for partnered sex and the ridges are meant to rub against a woman's clitoris during intercourse in certain positions. Once you have it on, move the textured part to the top so that it's facing up toward you. In general, they work best with face-to-face positions where you have close contact, such as Missionary, Cowgirl, and Yab-Yum.

Before you put on a nonadjustable ring, lube up both your penis and your balls to make getting the ring on smoother and easier. A cock ring is easier to put on when you're semi-hard, so warm yourself up a bit or ask your partner to, then step back and put the ring on. If you're hairy, be mindful that the ring can easily catch on your pubic hair and be careful. The best way to do it is to hold the ring just in front of your balls. First slip the skin of the scrotum through the ring. Next, slip one ball, then the other, through the ring, then push the head of your penis down and

slide your entire shaft through the ring. Follow this up with a nice hand job, blow job (or another kind of stimulation that gets you going), and feel the ring start to tighten as your erection grows. It should feel noticeably tight but never like it's cutting off all circulation. Never wear a cock ring for more than 15 or 20 minutes.

Adjustable Cock Rings: Easier to Use, Better Fit

Adjustable cock rings are easier to put on, adjust, and fit. They can be made of leather, neoprene, or rubber and usually have Velcro or snaps ($10 to $25). Neoprene is a synthetic rubber that's extremely resilient, can be used with all kinds of lube, and is easy to clean. These rings are easier to put on than their nonadjustable counterparts, because you simply wrap the strip around the base of the penis and balls, then snap or Velcro it closed. Men find that they can put them on when they are soft or semi-hard and adjust the tightness as their erection grows.

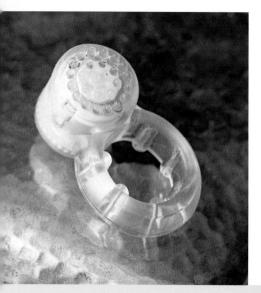

Iconic Ring

Vibrating Cock Rings: Something for Him *and* Her

Vibrating cock rings ($7 to $25) come in several different designs and work especially well during vaginal intercourse. Some vibrating rings have a vibrator built in, such as the silicone and rechargeable Bo by Tantus ($75 to $80). Most have a sheath or strap on top that houses a mini bullet vibrator. When you put one on, you should make sure the vibrator sits on top facing you, so that as you penetrate her vagina, the vibrator stimulates the tops of the base of your penis as well as her clitoris. Like the cock rings with textured nubs, vibrating rings work best in positions where you have close contact. Some women find that using a vibrating cock ring in positions that offer a lot of thrusting is just frustrating because one second the vibrator is against their clitoris and the next second it's gone. Positions like Horizontal Missionary, Coital Alignment Technique (CAT), Cowgirl (where she grinds against you), and Yab-Yum—which emphasize penetration with a rocking motion that keeps your bodies connected rather than traditional in-and-out thrusting—work much better. Alone or with a partner, you can also turn the vibrator around so it sits at the bottom and vibrates against the scrotum.

If you want to give or get the best of both worlds, check out the double vibrator cock rings, which have a vibrating bullet on each end. With the Twin Rabbit Cock Ring vibe ($25), you can wear it with one vibrator on top and the other on the bottom to stimulate her clitoris and her perineum. Or face the rabbits toward you for vibration against your shaft and scrotum.

Perfect Pairing: Iconic Ring + Horizontal Missionary Position

In Horizontal Missionary position, she lies on her back and he kneels between her legs. As he penetrates her vagina, he leans forward until he is lying completely on top of her. He can even kick his legs out behind him so that their bodies are completely parallel. A position like this is intimate and encourages intense pelvic rocking during penetration rather than frenzied thrusting. Because their pelvises stay so connected, this is a perfect position for a vibrating cock ring. The Iconic Ring by Jimmyjane ($36) is a high-quality elastomer cock ring with a small but powerful vibrator on top. The elastomer makes the ring stretchy and comfortable for him to put on and wear. The vibrator is encased in a textured sleeve with nubs that will feel great rubbing against her clitoris.

Metal cock rings look really cool but have no give to them whatsoever, so you need to be sure about the proper size before playing with one. My suggestion is to experiment with rubber rings to find the best diameter for you, then buy a metal ring. You can find a wide selection of cock rings with lots of bells and whistles at stores that cater to BDSM players and fetish enthusiasts. If you find that you really enjoy cock rings, you may want to see some of the more advanced and elaborate designs, including double cock rings (where one ring goes over your shaft and the other over your balls), locking cock rings, rings with leashes (for bondage and role-play), and designer cock rings made of stainless steel and even bronze.

Advanced Cock Rings: Size Matters

Metal cock rings look really cool but have no give to them whatsoever, so you need to be sure about the proper size before playing with one. My suggestion is to experiment with rubber rings to find the best diameter for you, then buy a metal ring. You can find a wide selection of cock rings with lots of bells and whistles at stores that cater to BDSM players and fetish enthusiasts. If you find that you really enjoy cock rings, you may want to see some of the more advanced and elaborate designs, including double cock rings (where one ring goes over your shaft and the other over your balls), locking cock rings, rings with leashes (for bondage and role-play), and designer cock rings made of stainless steel and even bronze.

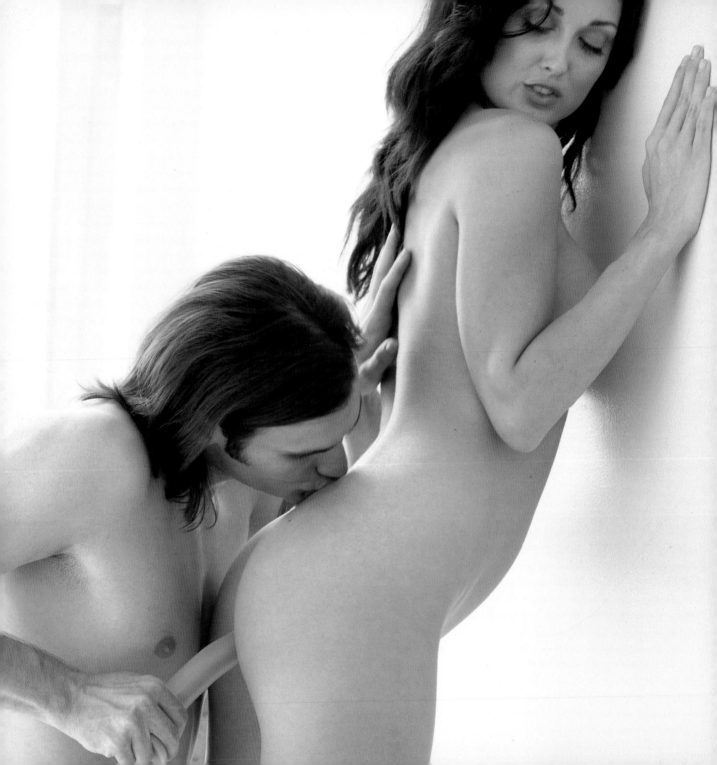

CHAPTER 14

DELICIOUS DILDOS AND WONDERFUL WANDS

Dildos and wands are insertable toys designed for penetration that don't vibrate. They come in a variety of materials, including rubber, softened PVC, vinyl, TPR, silicone, acrylic, glass, metal, and wood. They vary in length and width and can be as modest as the size of a finger or as grand as a tall soda can.

Some dildos are made to look like penises, while others are simply phallic in shape. Wands tend to have phallic, curvy, and creative shapes. Most dildos of soft materials were made to be compatible with dildo harnesses, so you can use them with your hand or strap them on if you wish. Wands are for handheld use.

A common question I get asked is, "If there's a penis in the room, why would you need or want a dildo?" Dildos are not meant to substitute for the penis, they are meant to complement the penis! Plenty of couples use dildos for all kinds of sex play. Some women like to put on a show, and being able to do themselves with a dildo in front of their partners is a big turn-on. Guys, pay attention! By watching her closely, you could learn something about what turns her on and how she likes to be penetrated; you can use this information later to your advantage and practice her penetration techniques with your penis.

Many couples like to play with a dildo before intercourse as a way to warm up for more penetration. If your partner is well endowed or you find intercourse painful or difficult at times, using a dildo that's about one size down from your partner's penis is a good way to get your vagina or ass open and ready for something bigger.

Or perhaps your partner's penis feels really good, but you crave more length or width, or both. Sometimes our bodies aren't always a perfect fit. After pregnancy, some women find their vaginas feel looser or crave something bigger to fill them. Women should never feel bad about their changing bodies; embrace the change, ladies. Whether your body has changed or not, obviously, a desire for something longer or thicker is a delicate, tricky subject to bring up. Many men are sensitive about the size of their penis or they worry they aren't big enough. Don't make it about comparison or competition. It's not about one being better than the other: You simply want both!

Maybe your partner often comes before you, but you want to keep going. Or perhaps when his penis is done for the night, you're just getting started. Using a dildo is one way for men to keep up with their multiorgasmic partners without taking Viagra. Some women love to have their G-spots stimulated and have wonderful G-spot orgasms, but intercourse just isn't the best way to get to their G-spot. A curved dildo or wand made especially for G-spot stimulation to the rescue!

If your partner feels threatened or uneasy with dildo play, remind him that you want *him* to use the dildo on you, and without him, it won't be as much fun. Help him realize that a dildo isn't a cop-out, and sex does not always have to revolve around his penis. Guys, remember: A dildo may not be part of your body, but when it's on the end of your hand, you're still the one who's going to get the credit for showing your girl a great time. And take it from me: She will have a great time.

Don't forget that dildos aren't just for the ladies. Men who enjoy anal penetration can use dildos alone or with their partners. For more information about anal pleasure, read the next chapter. To read about strap-on sex, see chapter 16. These are just some examples of ways that couples incorporate dildo and wand play into their lovemaking, but the bottom line is this: They're lots of fun!

Choosing a Dildo: Tips for Success

If you recall from chapter 4, there are many different materials for dildos:

- Rubber, softened PVC: soft and pliable texture, inexpensive, many styles, including very realistic, usually contain phthalates, porous and harder to clean

- Elastomer, TPR: soft and pliable texture, good alternative to rubber and PVC, can be phthalate-free, less porous

- Silicone: soft to medium-firm texture, warms to body temperature, resilient, more expensive, easy to clean, not compatible with silicone lube

- Acrylic, glass, wood, metal: rock-hard texture, smooth and seamless surface, resilient, most expensive, easy to clean, compatible with all lubes

If you're buying your first dildo, you may want to choose an inexpensive one of rubber, softened PVC, or TPR; if you decide you like it, you can spend some more for a better material. If you want the best soft material on the market, then definitely pick silicone—and make sure it's medical-grade or platinum silicone. Although I've noted the range of textures for each material, realize that different manufacturers produce different textures. For example, a Doc Johnson jelly rubber toy will be softer and squishier than a California Exotics rubber toy. Tantus makes silicone dildos that tend to be firmer and less pliable than the silicone of Vixen Creations. VixSkin by Vixen Creations feels very similar to CyberSkin, but is easier to clean and lasts longer.

When it comes to aesthetics, you have a lot to choose from. If you want a dildo that most closely resembles the male member, you're more likely to find it in rubber, PVC, or thermal plastic; realistic dildos come in different skin tones, with balls, circumcised heads, and veins. If you want some realism, but can do without details like veins, you can find realistic silicone dildos as well, especially VixSkin by Vixen Creations. Perhaps

you're down with the shape, but don't need it to actually look like a cock to work for you. There are plenty of dildos that are phallic, but leave off any other references to penises. They're usually available in bright colors and can have interesting textures such as ridges or bumps. Maybe you want to get away from the penis altogether, and have a dildo that looks nothing like a dick. Well, you can do that, too. There are dildos fashioned to look like goddesses, sea creatures, animals, and even astrological signs.

You should decide in advance whether you'd like to use your dildo with your hands, in a strap-on harness, or both. If you want to strap it on, then choose a dildo with a flared base that is harness compatible; dildos without bases will not stay put when worn in a harness. If you're not sure, ask a salesperson. For more information on harnesses and strap-ons, see chapter 16.

Perfect Pairing: Vixen Mistress Dildo + Standing Position

Have her stand facing you and leaning up against a wall. Get down on your knees and begin teasing her with your mouth. Kiss her belly, her inner thighs, and her

hipbones. Venture to her outer labia and use the entire length of your tongue against one side, then the other. Move to her inner labia and use long strokes of the tongue like you're licking an ice cream cone. Dip a finger into her opening and spread her wetness around her vulva. Slide the finger back in as your mouth moves up to her clitoris. As you feel her get more turned on, add another finger. Have the Mistress dildo ($44) standing by for when she's ready. Pour some lube in your hand and coat the dildo. Take the head of the dildo and run it between her inner lips and up to her clit. Slide it between her lips a few times, then rub it against her clit. Let your fingers (or hers) take over rubbing her clit while you slowly slide the dildo inside her. Go about halfway, then stop and let it linger there while her body gets used to it. Push it in farther as you continue to play with her clitoris. Put your mouth back on her as you pump the dildo in and out of her. If you want, turn her around so she's facing the wall and ask her to present her ass to you. Slide the dildo in again, this time from behind, creating a different sensation.

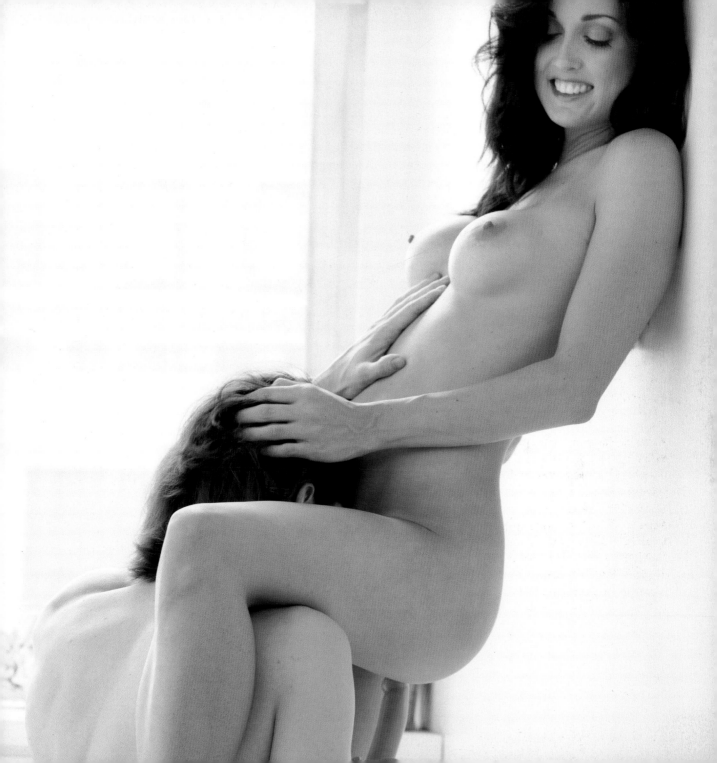

Other Types of Soft Dildos: Vibrations, Inflations, and More

Vibrating dildos: I just got done telling you that a dildo is an insertable toy that doesn't vibrate, and now, to throw a wrench in the mix . . . introducing vibrating dildos. What is the difference between a vibrator and a vibrating dildo? Vibrating dildos are harness-compatible dildos that have a hole in the base for a vibrating mini bullet. You can use the dildo with or without the vibrator. In fact, many companies make two versions of the same dildo: one with the hole and one without. For those folks who like penetration and vibration, look for a vibrating dildo.

Inflatable dildos: An inflatable dildo is a hollow sheath of rubber attached to a pump that inflates it. For people interested in working their way up in size who don't want to invest in multiple dildos, an inflatable dildo is a good alternative. Some people don't like them, however, because they don't feel solid like other dildos. Others enjoy the unique sensation they create: They can feel the toy expand while it's inside their vagina or ass.

Double-ended dildos: Double-ended dildos are perfect for couples where the man likes anal penetration and both partners want to enjoy simultaneous penetration. The traditional design—an extra-long dildo with a head on each end—is actually not very functional when it comes down to it. It's hard to use and often just doesn't work. The Feeldoe, distributed by Tantus ($115 to $150), is a silicone double dildo that actually works because it's not one long straight phallus, but rather two dildos joined together at a fulcrum; it was originally designed for lesbians to have dildo sex without a strap-on harness. One partner puts the short bulbous end inside her and she can actually use her body to penetrate the other partner with the longer end. This is by far one of the most popular toys in recent years, and though some have attempted to copy its unique design, the original stands alone. The Feeldoe comes with or without a bullet vibrator.

Choosing a Wand

Wands are insertable toys that can't be worn in a strap-on, and they are most often made of hard materials such as glass, metal, wood, acrylic, and hard plastic. Because of their high-quality materials, wands tend to be expensive, and many are over $100. Although some of them are straight phallic shapes, many of them are curved or shaped like a U or an S. Both their curved shape and their hard texture make wands ideal toys for G-spot and prostate (P-spot) stimulation. Many people find that a toy with a solid surface works much better than one made of a pliable material. This makes sense because both the G-spot and the P-spot respond to firm, deliberate pressure.

The Crystal Wand from Nectar Products ($55) was one of the first toys made of a hard material that departed from the phallic shape of most dildos and wands; introduced more than a decade ago, it's made of medical-grade acrylic and was designed with an exaggerated S shape by Tantra teacher Cynthia Lamborne. The shape made it easy to hold and maneuver and perfect for G-spot stimulation. The Crystal Wand is quite slim, so it's good for those who find other wands too big; the same company makes a prostate toy called the Crystal Wand Honeydipper, which is even slimmer.

Glass wands are as gorgeous as they are functional. With unique shapes, dazzling colors, and handmade quality, glass wands have become very popular in recent years. They are like individual works of art, and often their owners want to display them rather then squirrel them away under the bed! They can be fashioned to look like a penis, a baton, a curved wand, and even a candy cane! Some of the top glass toy brands include Phallix, Asstroknots, and XHale. Most well-stocked sex shops carry at least a few glass toys and several websites cater specifically to glass toy lovers. The website Blowfish.com has one of the best selections of glass dildos and wands on the Internet, and the buyer always selects some of the most unique pieces out there, many one-of-a-kind pieces made by local artisans and designers. The most important thing to know when buying a glass toy is that it's made of medical-grade borosilicate, which can withstand extreme heat and cold as well as pressure and shock; one of the most well-known brand names of this type of

glass is Pyrex. These toys are compatible with all kinds of lubricants, and lube clings nicely to the seamless surface. Some of my favorite glass toys are the Inside Out Filligrino G-Spot Shaft by Phallix ($300), the Juicer by Asstroknots ($100), and the Archer by E-Glass ($50).

Like glass, aluminum toys are striking in their modern, streamlined designs. They are smooth and shiny and are often heavier than glass wands. They are easy to clean, compatible with all lubes, and some of the best G-spot and P-spot toys

in the world. Njoy dominates the metal toy market with its ingeniously designed, brilliantly functional wands and anal toys. Its best seller is the S-shaped Fun Wand ($88); one end has three teardrop-shaped balls and the other end has a single ball on the end. The Pure Wand ($108) is thicker than the Fun Wand and has a smooth, curvy U shape. Tantus, known for its silicone toys, launched the Alumina line of aluminum toys; these toys are much lighter than those Njoy makes.

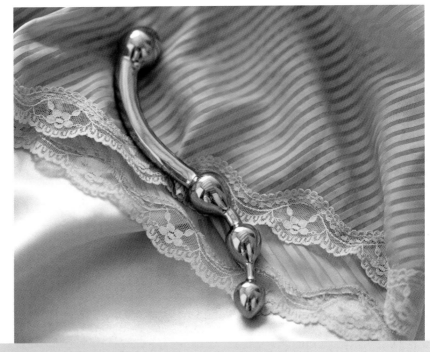

Fun Wand

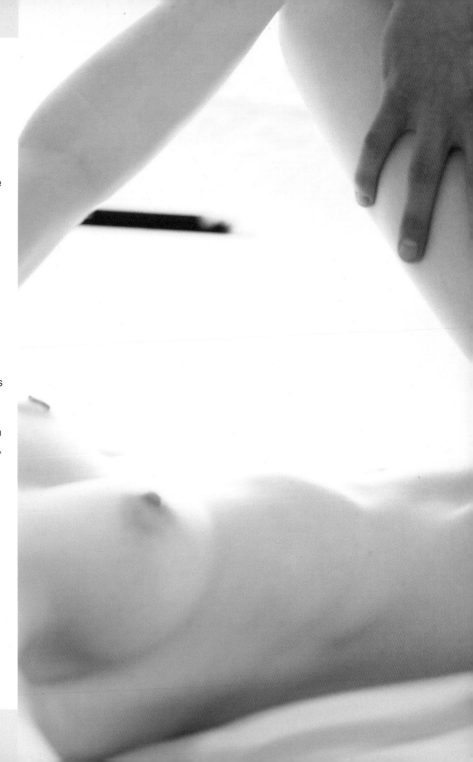

Perfect Pairing: Fun Wand + Flying Missionary Position

In Flying Missionary position, she lies on her back with her butt scooted down to the edge of the bed, and he stands at the edge of the bed. She bends her knees and rests her feet on his abdomen. The success of this position depends on the height of your bed, of course. Warm her up with some oral sex or manual stimulation, and when she's ready, slide the well-lubed Fun Wand inside her. Start with the one-ball end and aim the curved end toward the front of her body to stimulate her G-spot. She should feel the ball press against her G-spot as the toy moves in and out of her. This position has many of the pluses of Missionary position—it's good for eye contact, communication, and kissing. Women can take a more active role in the penetration, using their feet for leverage to push off their partner's body. He has lots of thrusting power because he is standing, and both partners have a great view of each other's bodies.

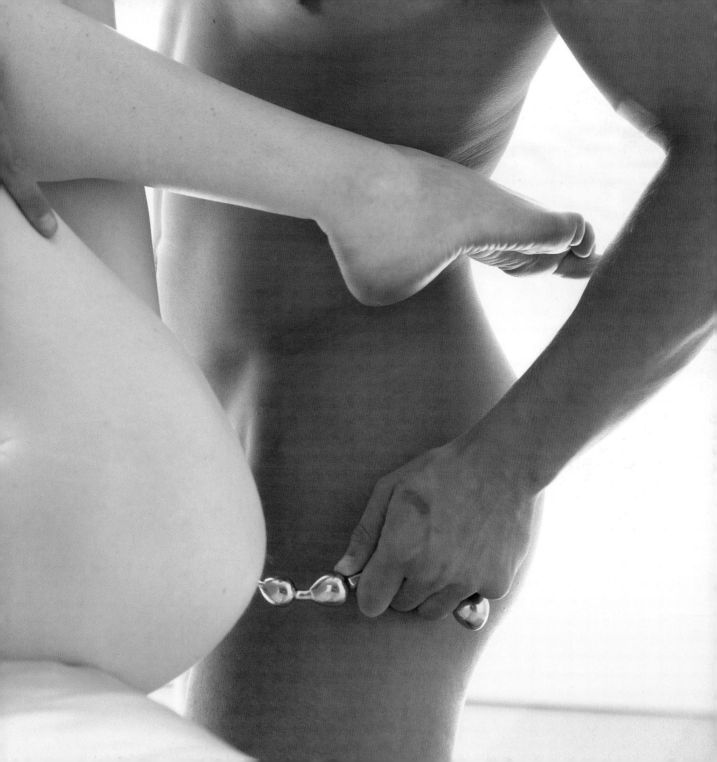

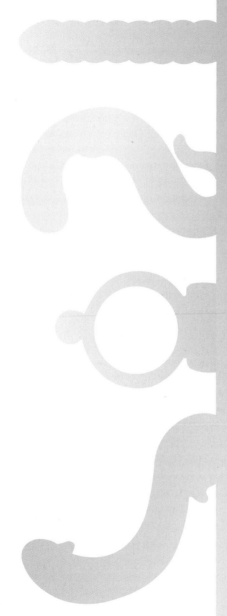

You're Worth the Splurge: Luxury Wand

Australian-based company Goldfrau makes beautiful handcrafted ceramic wands ($220 to $240) that are as much sculptures as they are sex toys (available at Good Vibrations). Each one comes in two sizes of the same shape—a slim, straight phallic shape with a round ball on one end meant to be the handle—and it comes in several designs, embellished with intricate, colorful patterns and images. Run it under warm water for a few minutes and you've got a smooth, warm, seamless toy that can stand up against any glass or metal dildo.

NobEssence makes sculptural, ergonomic wands (dildos and cock rings, too) of wood—exotic hardwoods including cocobolo, bamboo, bloodwood, and macassare ebony—all organic and sustainably farmed for those of you who worry about depleting our forests ($100 to $250). Each toy is a handcrafted masterpiece, but they're not just nice to look at! The toys are hypoallergenic and sealed in a sixteen-step finishing process with Lubrosity (a trade-secret coating), making them waterproof, safe for penetration, and easy to clean. With clever shapes and body-conscious curves, the toys are perfect for G-spot and P-spot stimulation.

Your Guide to Using Dildos and Wands

Some women like penetration while they masturbate some of the time or all of the time. If you've tried insertable vibrators but are looking for something softer, more pliable, or that looks and feels more like a penis, you may want to try a dildo. If you want something firmer and more angled for the G-spot, then a wand may be the perfect tool for the job.

Always use plenty of lube on the dildo—remember, it will feel much better inside you when it's slick and rarin' to go! Whether you are alone or with a partner, start slow and tease with the dildo; rub it on the outside of the vaginal opening, against the labia and clitoris. Start penetration with a well-lubed finger or two to get your body warmed up and ready for something bigger. Along with the dildo, you may want to add clitoral stimulation—your partner can go down on you, rub your clit with his fingers, or use a vibrator on you. Clitoral stimulation will feel great and help your vagina relax, expand, and be ready for the dildo. Never just shove a dildo inside; there will be plenty of time for fast and furious later on, but in the beginning it's best to be slow, methodical, and gentle.

To use a curved dildo or wand for G-spot stimulation, make sure the curve is aimed toward the navel. Remember, a light touch just won't do much for the G-spot. You want to strive for deliberate, direct pressure. The key, as with other kinds of stimulation, is to build the intensity; don't go too hard too quickly. Communicate with your partner and see what feels best for her. You can experiment with different techniques. For example, apply an equal amount of pressure and movement. Some women like a lot of pressure and only a little movement. Other women like a lot of movement where you're stimulating the G-spot as you move the toy in and out with long strokes. Experiment with how much pressure, penetration, and movement she likes—ask her which techniques feel the best to her. While you're so diligently focused on the G-spot, don't forget about the clitoris! Some women prefer G-spot stimulation by itself, while others appreciate both at once. Because all the nerves and tissues are connected, they play off one other, helping stimulate the entire area.

Top Dildo and Wand Brands

See Resource Guide (page 238) for more information

Realistic dildos:
Vixen Creations VixSkin line

Harness-compatible dildos:
Vixen Creations, Tantus Silicone

Handheld dildos and wands:
Jollies, Njoy, Nob Essence, Phallix

Tristan's Top Picks: Double and Simultaneous Penetration Toys

For women who like to have both orifices penetrated at the same time or couples who want to experience simultaneous penetration, these are toys designed to double your fun.

Pipedreams Lucky Lady Blue Dolphin ($15 to $20): This phthalate-free rubber dildo is curved in a U shape for simultaneous anal and vaginal penetration.

Devinn Lane's Double Action by Swedish Erotica ($25 to $35): This phallic-style vibrator has two smooth phallic shafts that vibrate.

Sportsheets Menage-a-Trois Harness ($50): If your partner wants to be able to penetrate you in both places at once, try this strap-on harness with two holes, one for a penis (or dildo) for the vagina and another for a penis (or dildo) for the ass.

Feeldoe ($115 to $150): For couples who want to experience penetration at the same time without the use of a strap-on harness, the Feeldoe is the perfect toy. One partner slides the smaller, knobby end inside him or her, then the longer phallic end goes inside the other partner.

Double Penetration: Pleasure Times Two

Lots of women love the feeling of having both vaginal and anal penetration simultaneously. Some even fantasize about having two penises at the same time. If you are interested in experiencing double penetration without having a threesome with another man, a dildo can definitely get that job done! One penis plus one dildo can equal two happy holes.

The trick for double penetration is to use lots and lots of lube, go slow, and work your way up to it. Communication is extremely important: You're testing the limits of her body here, so make sure she's giving you plenty of feedback about how it feels. Also realize that some women can easily and comfortably accommodate something of size in their vagina and in their ass. Others will take some effort, with lots of warm-up. But some women may not be able to do it at all, and you should never pressure her to try it if it's just not working. Double penetration really depends on your internal map and whether there's room for two. Most women will have an idea whether it's possible, so make sure she's the one who's in charge and calling the shots. Some women like to first have their ass fully penetrated by their partner's penis (because that orifice takes more time to warm up), then have a dildo slowly slid into their vagina. Others prefer the inching method, where the penis inches into the vagina a little at a time and stays put, then the dildo inches into the ass a little, and so on. Remember, you can also do this with two small dildos if his penis is too big, impatient, or out of commission.

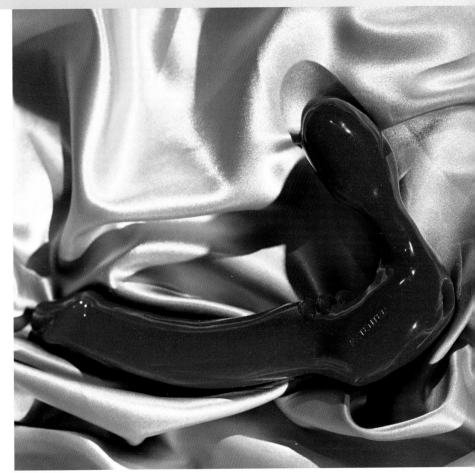

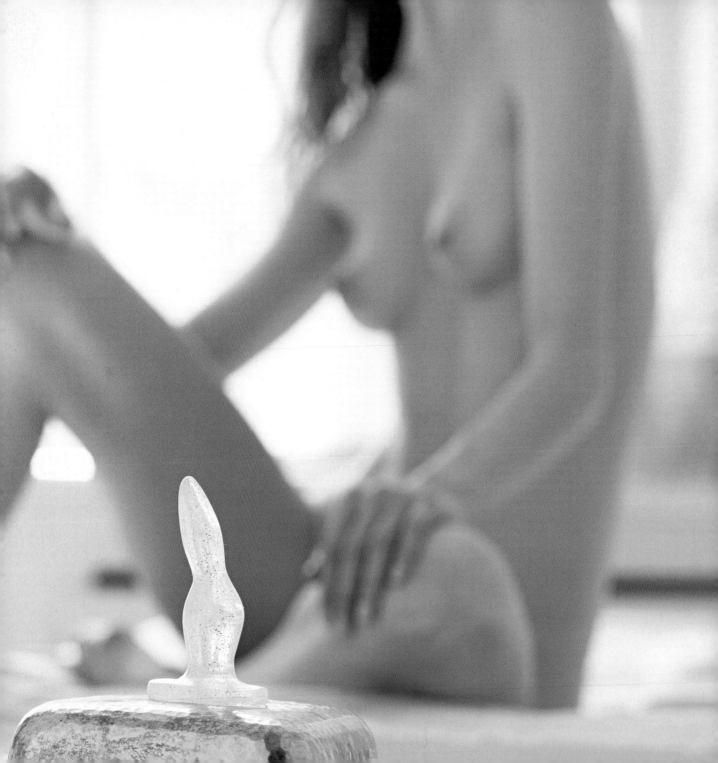

CHAPTER 15

ANAL PLEASURE:
Butt Toys for Her and Him

As you read in the first chapter, the ass is an amazing erogenous zone. Women can have orgasms from anal penetration, in combination with vaginal penetration or clitoral stimulation, or on its own. Men can achieve direct prostate stimulation through anal penetration, which, by itself or coupled with penis stimulation, can also lead to orgasm. It's important to talk to your partner about anal play before you do it, and keep communicating while you explore.

The ass is not self-lubricating, so you absolutely need to use lube, and plenty of it. The key to safe, pleasurable anal sex is slow, patient warm-up. The biggest mistake people make is that they rush the process, which leads to pain and frustration. Anal sex does not have to hurt; if it hurts, you need to slow down or stop altogether.

Toys are a great way to explore anal pleasure on your own, experiment with your partner, or warm up for anal intercourse. A toy must have either a handle or a flared base to be safe for anal play (so slimline, rabbit-style, or straight phallic vibrators should not be used). Some vibrators and most dildos and wands are safe for your ass; in addition, there are toys designed especially for anal pleasure.

Anal Beads: Fun Going in, Fun Coming Out

Anal beads come in many different varieties. One particular style used to be the most abundant and inexpensive: hard plastic beads on a nylon or cotton string. If you see those, steer clear of them: they are cheaply made, impossible to clean properly, and potentially unsafe (because the plastic usually has rough edges or seams). You want to look for an anal bead toy, which is one continuous piece of rubber or silicone. I recommend silicone, because it warms to body temperature and can be easily disinfected. Some bead toys have beads that are all the same size and others graduate in size; pick a size and style that appeals to you.

What fans of anal beads love about them is the ability to experience one particular sensation several times over—when the sphincter muscles relax, the anus opens up, a bead slides in, and the muscles close around it. (Some toys have five beads, others as many as ten.) Make sure you lube each part of the bead toy and go slowly as you insert each part. The fun thing about them is that once you have a portion or the entire length of the beads in your ass, you can pull the toy out all at once, creating an entirely different sensation! Some people like to pull it out just before orgasm, to push them over the edge, while others wait until after they've come.

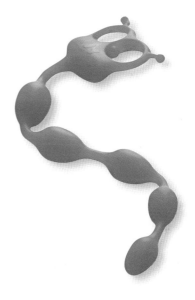

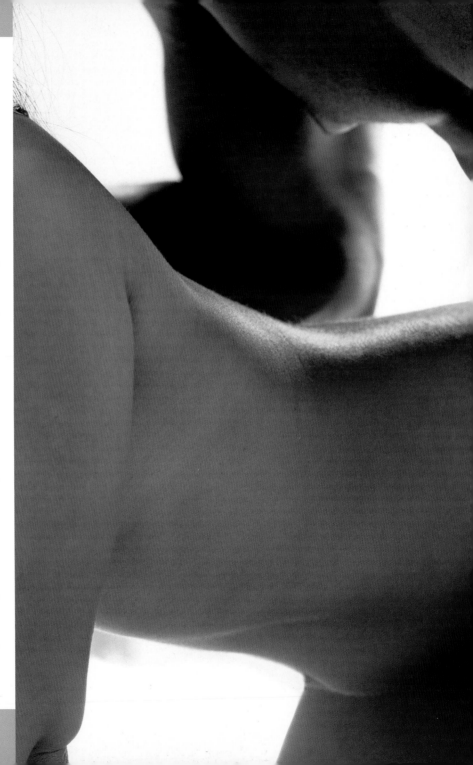

Perfect Pairing: Flexi Felix Beads + Stallion Position

In Stallion position, she stands with her legs apart, then bends forward at the waist and leans on the bed (or another piece of furniture) and he stands behind her. Stallion has all the benefits of Doggie Style with more power, because he has full leverage with his hips and legs. For some couples, this may simply work better than Doggie Style or Flying Doggie because of their sizes and heights. If she feels too much strain on her knees in other Doggie positions, this is a better option for her. If he can position his hips slightly higher than hers, he can stimulate her G-spot indirectly when he penetrates her.

Once you're inside her vagina, lube up Fun Factory's Flexi Felix bead toy ($35). It's a great toy because it's soft silicone and the beads are small—perfect for a beginner. Slide one bead inside her anus, and let her ass relax and get used to the feeling. Have her rub her clitoris as you do it to intensify the sensations. Ask her when she's ready for the next bead, then slide that one in gently. See how many beads she can take, but don't press your luck, everyone has to go at her own pace. Hold the handle of the toy, then start to thrust gently inside her. As you move inside her, the beads will feel even tighter.

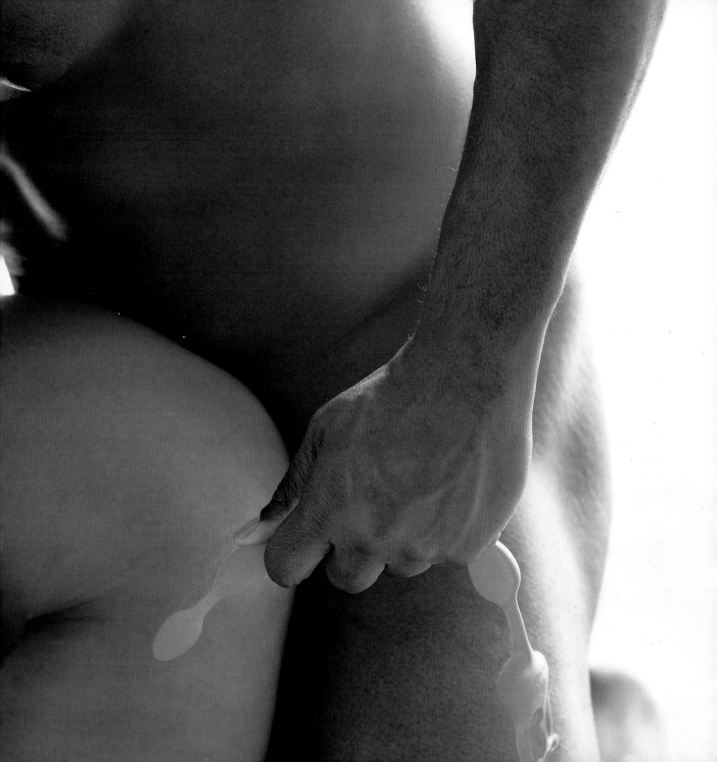

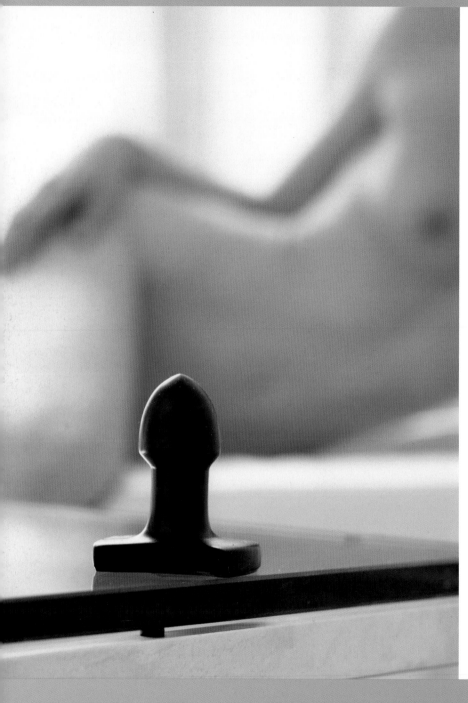

Butt Plugs: Great for Solo Play or as a Warm-up to Anal Intercourse

Butt plugs are made especially for anal play, and are made of rubber, PVC, hard plastic, TPR, silicone, glass, acrylic, metal, and wood. They are designed to go in your ass and stay there. It's a deceptively simple concept, but one that is very gratifying for a lot of people. Plugs come in a variety of styles and materials, but most stick to a few basic shapes. The classic teardrop plug is tapered at the top, is pear shaped in the middle with a well-defined wide part, has a very slim neck underneath for the sphincter to close around, and has a round or an oval base at the bottom. The bubble or ripple style usually has multiple bubble-shaped sections (in the same size or graduated sizes) that descend into the narrow neck and flared base. The mushroom-shaped plug has a thick mushroom cap head, a neck that's narrower than the head but not as narrow as on the other two styles, and an oval-shaped base.

The Tristan Silicone Butt Plug

For those folks who like the feeling of having something in their ass—a sensation of fullness, "stretching," or pressure—without any in-and-out movement, a butt plug is the ideal toy. Unless the plug is the size of one finger, you always want to warm up with a finger or two before inserting it. Make sure it is well lubed and never push too hard or force it inside. Take your time. Ease it all the way in and feel the sphincter muscles close around the neck.

Butt plugs are great for solo play as well as perfect tools for warm-up to anal penetration. Some people like to slide a butt plug in, then move on to other activities such as oral sex, vaginal penetration, or mutual masturbation. After the plug has been in for a little while, slide it out and you'll find the ass is aroused, open, and ready for something bigger.

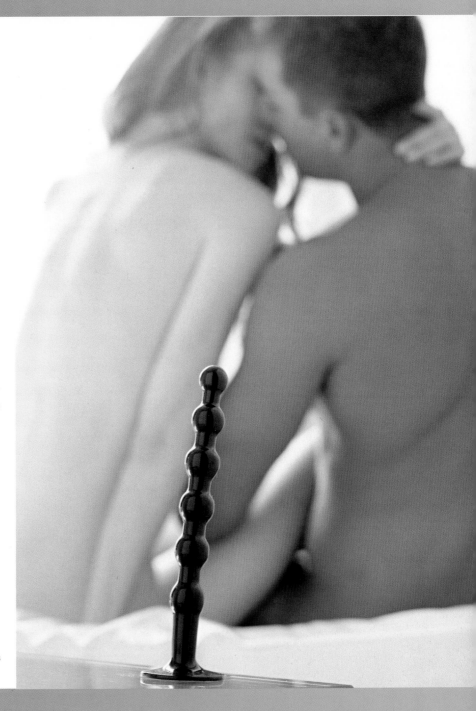

Tanutus Silicone Anal Beads

An inflatable butt plug is just what it sounds like: a hollow plug (usually made of latex) attached to a bulb you squeeze with your hand to push air into and inflate it. Some inflatable butt plugs also have vibrators in their bases. Some people like inflatable plugs because they can gradually work their way up from a slim toy to a sizable one without having to shell out the money for four different-sized plugs! They can track their progress, and one toy can suit their different desires. Other people like the unique feeling of something expanding while it's inside their ass. As with all kinds of anal play, don't try to rush things with this kind of toy—take your time. Use common sense and never overinflate one of these bad boys. Make sure you first inflate it outside the body, and note how many squeezes of the inflating pump it can take, because you don't want to find out its limit while it's up your butt.

For some people, if it doesn't vibrate, it doesn't do the trick, and these folks swear by vibrating anal toys. Vibration not only feels good, but it's also a proven way to relax muscles, so vibrating toys are great for anal penetration. There are butt plugs with attached vibrators and those that come with a removable vibrator so you can have the best of both worlds. There are vibrating probes made and marketed especially for anal play. Some not only vibrate but are also bendable to allow for the perfect angle.

I recommend plugs made of soft materials for beginners, but when you're ready for something solid, some of the best plugs out there are made of glass, metal, and wood. Butt toys made of hard materials are smooth and seamless, and lube clings to them very well. Because there is no drag like on a soft toy, people often find they can take a bigger toy made of a hard material. For folks who really enjoy a feeling of fullness, the weight of one of these toys (especially the metal ones) totally satisfies.

Perfect Pairing: Buddy Plug + Reverse Cowgirl Position

In Reverse Cowgirl position, he usually lies on his back, but this time he should sit up. She straddles him facing away from him. Lube up the Buddy Plug (a great small plug from Vixen Creations, $18) and hold it underneath her. Have her take a deep breath and sit down on the plug so that she can control the speed and depth of the penetration. When it's securely inside her butt, you want to leave it there and give her body a chance to warm up. In this position, you can slide your penis inside her vagina while the plug is in her ass. Or she can slide her body back for some delicious oral sex in 69 position. Or she can reverse direction—for a blow job or intercourse in Cowgirl position. If she stays in Reverse Cowgirl, you can replace the Buddy with a bigger plug. Once she's had the bigger one in for a while, slide it out. Re-lube your penis, and have her come down slowly on it, like she did with the plug. This way, she's in charge of how much she takes and she can ride you exactly how she wants.

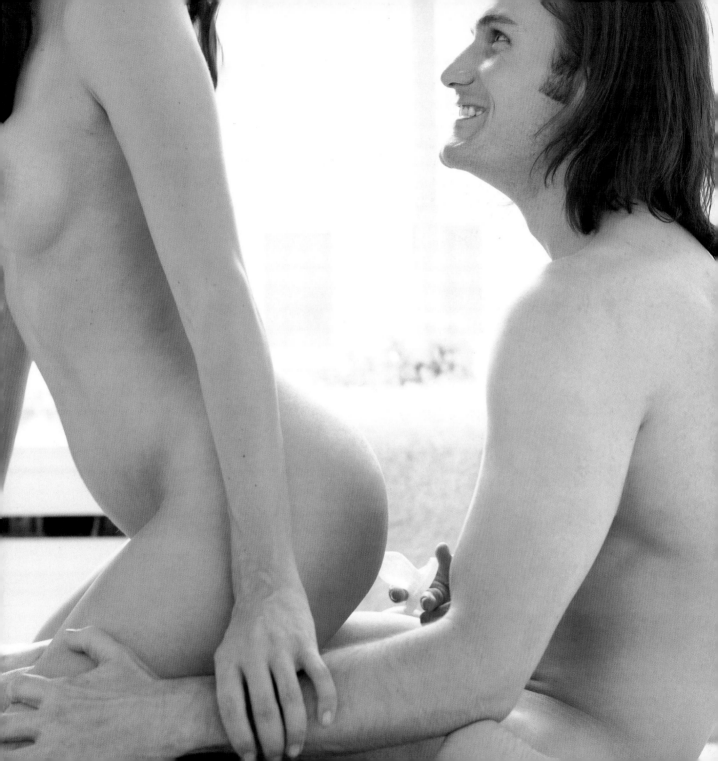

Perfect Pairing: Pure Plug + Triple X Position

To get into Triple X position, he lies on his back with his legs spread slightly. (Use pillows to make sure you're in a comfortable position.) She climbs on top of him and begins in Reverse Cowgirl position. Very slowly, she leans forward, letting her legs fall open, until she's lying on her stomach on top of and away from him. This is an advanced position and may not work for everyone, especially if it puts too much strain on his penis. In Triple X, he gets a great view of her ass and easy access to it as well. Njoy's Pure Plug ($65 to $120) comes in four sizes; after you've mastered two fingers, you're ready for the medium ($75). There are two ways to do this. The first is where there is no vaginal penetration; she simply lies on top of you. You can lube up the Pure Plug and slowly slide it into her ass. As you come to the widest part of the plug, have her take some very deep breaths. If you're having trouble, she can bear down slightly (as if she's pushing something out of her ass), which will help relax the sphincter muscles. Once the plug is all the way in, slip a compact clitoral vibrator underneath her and she'll be squirming in no time! The second version has her riding your penis in Reverse Cowgirl, then gradually leaning forward toward your feet. While you are still inside her, slide the well-lubed plug into her ass. The combination of both holes being filled at once should send her into ecstasy.

You're Worth the Splurge: Luxury Butt Plug

French artist Julian Snelling (juliansnelling.fr) designs butt plugs that look like jewelry. These stainless steel teardrop-shaped plugs range in size, but even the largest is fairly small. When you slide the plug inside someone's ass, that's when you see the crowning jewel—literally. On the base of each plug is a gorgeous, sparkling crystal. A plug with a colored crystal looks like a gorgeous ruby or emerald nestled between your partner's ass cheeks, quite a sight to behold! He also makes plugs with semiprecious stones, including malachite and tigereye, as well as some with intricate designs in bronze ($85 to $425).

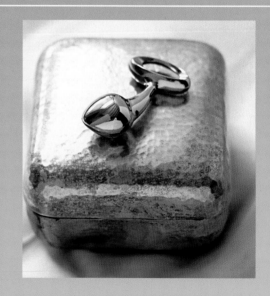

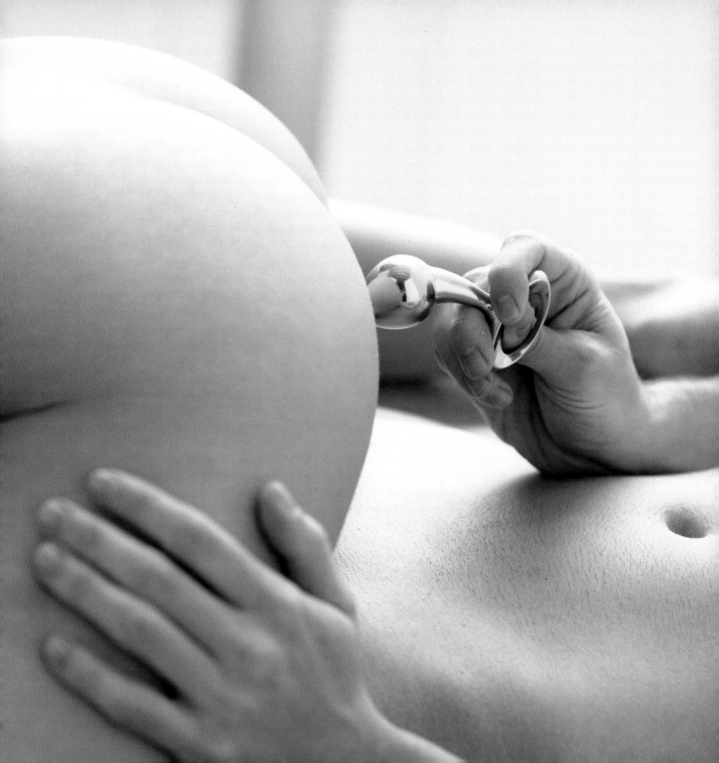

You're Worth the Splurge: Jade Butt Plug at Coco de Mer

For the anal aficionado who has every butt toy imaginable, surprise her with Petite Fesse ($140), a plug made of jade. Jade has long been associated with love and sexuality, and it's rare to find sex toys made of this precious stone. When you slide the plug all the way in your ass, the base that is nestled between the butt cheeks is a delicately carved flower.

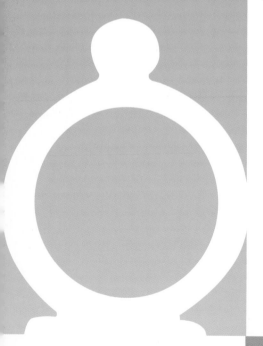

Prostate Toys: His Treat

Several sex toys have been designed especially for prostate stimulation. The Aneros was the very first prostate toy on the market, and it was originally created as a medical device to help men with swollen or enlarged prostates. It is made of nonporous hard plastic and looks like a butt plug with two curlicue ends on it. Men discovered that not only did it help them, but it also brought them tremendous pleasure and enhanced their orgasms. It has been embraced as a tool of pleasure and the brand has expanded as a result: The Aneros now comes in seven different styles.

There are now several prostate toys on the market, which all follow the basic premise of the Aneros toys: They are hands-free prostate stimulators. Slide the well-lubed toy inside your ass and its shape conforms to the inside of your body and targets the sensitive prostate internally and the perineum externally. As you tighten your sphincter muscles, the toy presses against the prostate; as you relax the muscles, the outer piece (which is different on different toys) stimulates your perineum. Not only do prostate toys massage the prostate, but they also help men tone and control their anal sphincter and PC muscles—which has been proven to improve sexual function and orgasm control and intensity.

Romp by NobEssence

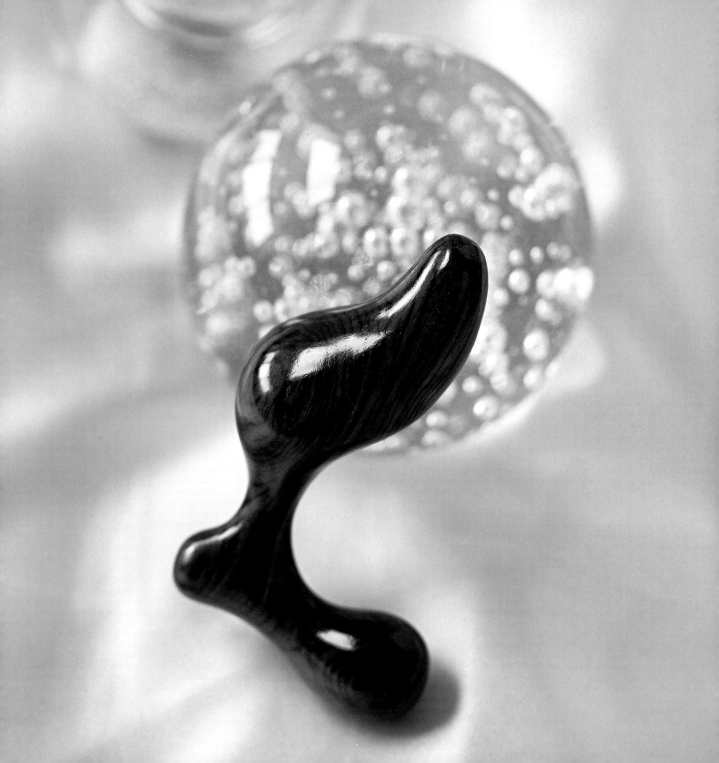

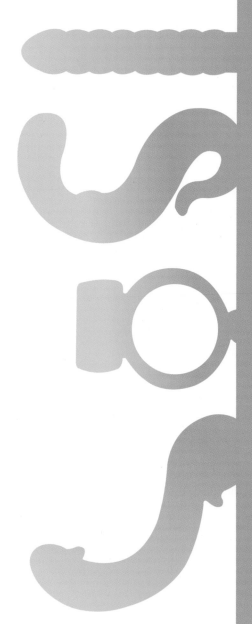

Tristan's Top Picks: Prostate Massagers

Aneros ($48 to $100): The original prostate massager brand still dominates the market and earns rave reviews from men all over the world. Start with the most popular style called MGX ($48). As you move your sphincter muscles it causes the toy to pivot forward to massage the prostate as the outer piece (called the abutment) rubs against the perineum.

Nexus Vibro: Nexus, a company based in the UK, makes several prostate toys, including Glide ($55), Excel ($60), Titus ($75), and a vibrating version called the Vibro ($120). Nexus toys are made of hard, nonporous plastic and have a similar shape to the Aneros, but with a more exaggerated angle. One of the significant differences is that instead of a thin piece of plastic to stimulate the perineum, Nexus toys have a stainless steel roller ball that glides against the sensitive spot (and the ball pops out for easy cleaning).

Rude Boy ($85): Created by the makers of the Rock Chick (which you read about in the chapter on dual-action vibrators), the Rude Boy is a silicone U-shaped, battery-powered, waterproof vibrator. The smooth part goes inside your ass, and its dramatic curve targets the sensitive prostate, while the end with raised nubs hugs your perineum. Like other prostate massagers, this is designed for hands-free fun: As you contract your sphincter muscles, the toy stimulates the prostate and perineum simultaneously.

Pfun Plug ($90): Njoy makes the best stainless steel toys in the world, period. They have ingenious, functional designs that really work, as though they've been tested on real bodies, not just made to look nice. The craftsmanship is top rate, and they come in luxurious satin-lined boxes like the small works of art that they are. The Pfun Plug has a curved shape and is the perfect length to hit the prostate. You can manually move it in and out with the cool ringed handle at the base or use your sphincter muscles to control it and let the base rub against the perineum. If you're looking for a toy with more weight than the others or you like stainless steel, nothing beats the Pfun.

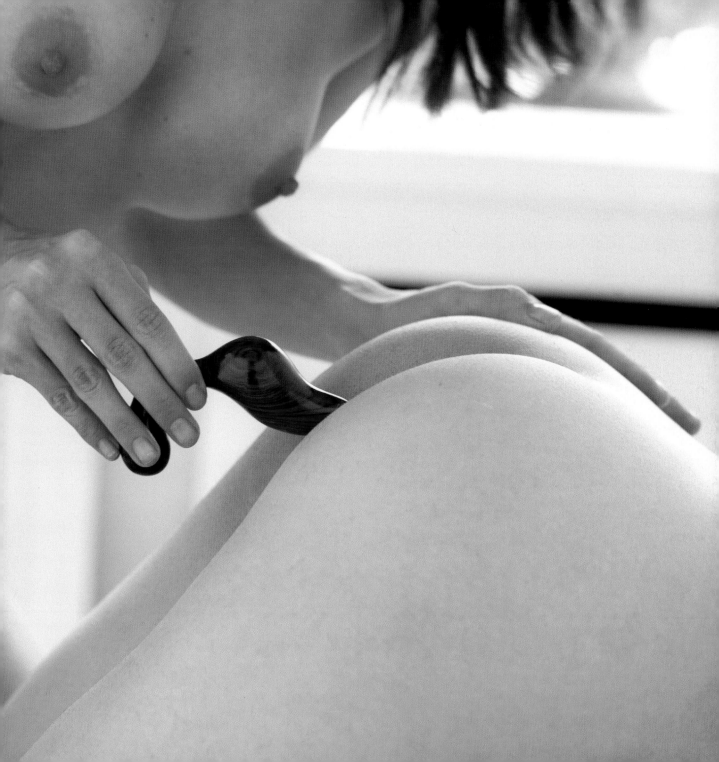

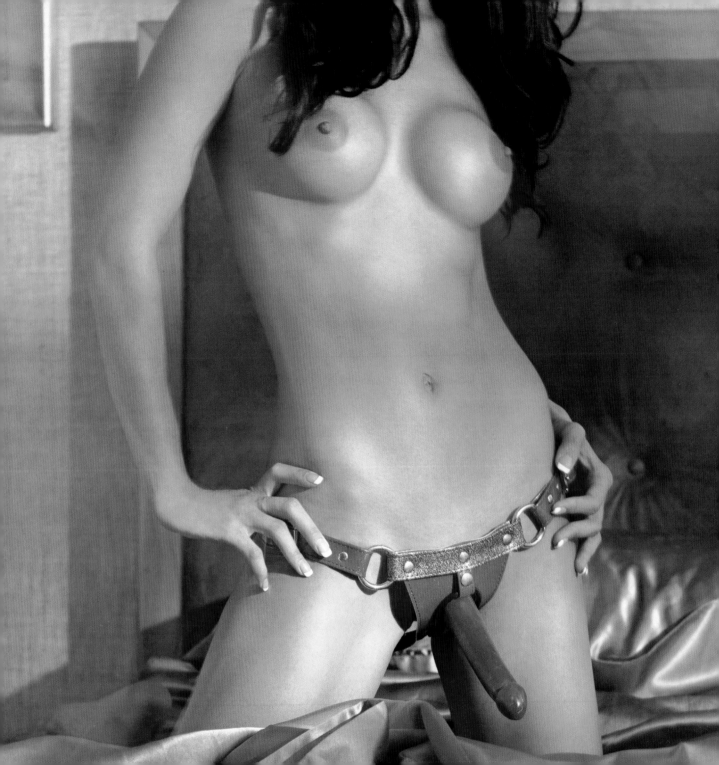

CHAPTER 16

GET READY FOR THE RIDE OF YOUR LIFE:

Strap-ons

Strap-ons are a great way to experience penetrative sex. Women can strap on a dildo to give their partners anal penetration. Men can strap on a dildo to give their partners vaginal or anal penetration, or both. Dildos and harnesses mean that you can have a hands-free romp and use your hands for other things: play with his balls, tweak her nipples, grab his butt cheeks. People also like the closeness a strap-on affords partners during penetration. Having strap-on sex can be part of fantasy role-playing or gender play for some partners.

It gives women the opportunity to learn a new way to give pleasure by having a dick. It's also a chance for couples to incorporate a sex toy into their bedroom routine in a new way.

A Thigh Harness Lets You Get Creative

A thigh harness is a piece of material (either stretchy nylon, neoprene, or leather) that you strap onto your leg. Neoprene gets the best reviews because it stays put—no one wants a harness that slips! It has a hole for a dildo to slip through and is usually kept in place by Velcro. Dildos without balls or very thick bases work best with this kind of harness. Thigh harnesses are great for people who don't want to wear a dildo between their legs, but still want to have hands-free dildo sex. If you like to rub up against your partner's thigh or love positions where you're on top, you'll also like a thigh harness, because you can climb on and ride to your heart's content! Although it was designed to be worn on your leg, you're also free to get creative. Strap it to a firm pillow or the base of a chair for solo play. Rap it around your partner's arms for bondage and dildo play all in one.

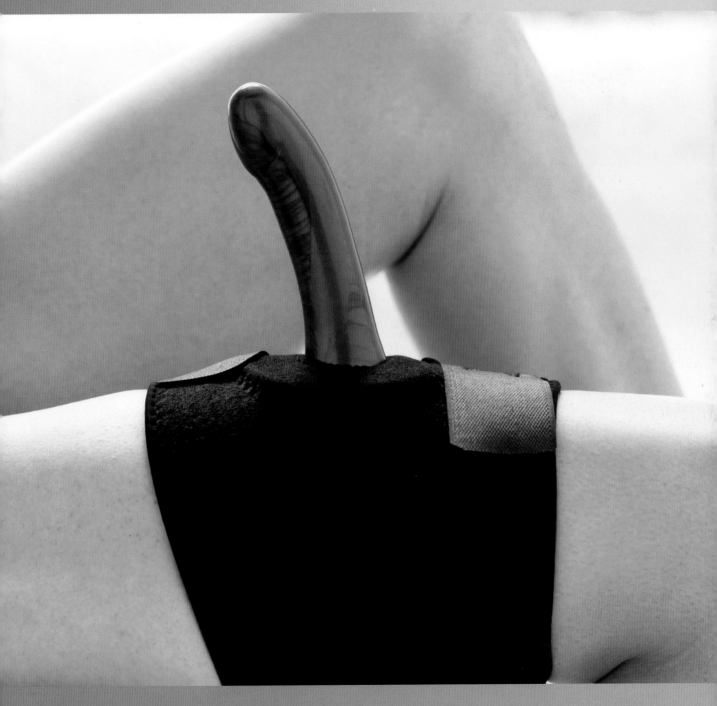

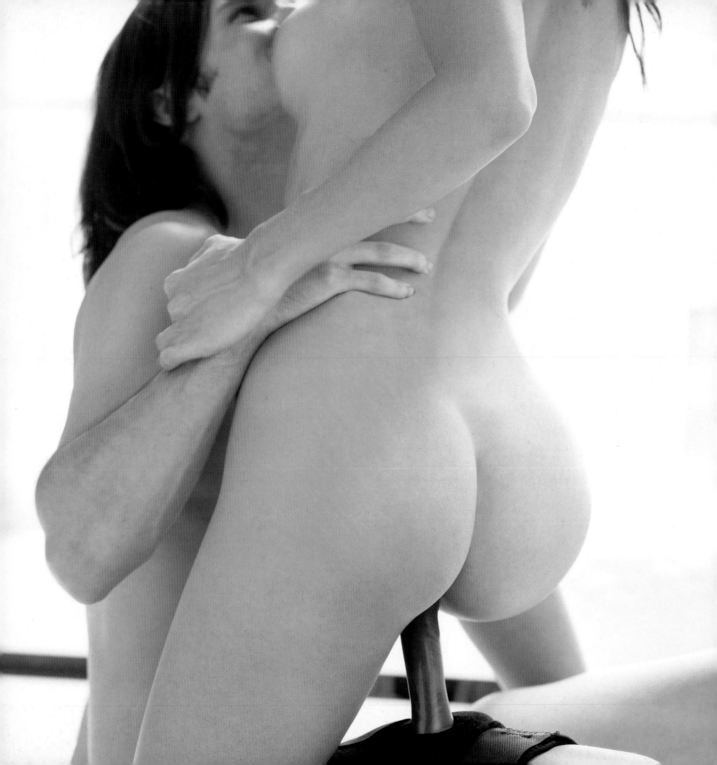

Perfect Pairing: Thigh Harness + Froggie Position

Have him lie on his back with the harness and dildo strapped to one thigh. Climb on top to straddle him, but instead of resting on your knees, squat down, so your feet are flat. Begin by teasing him a little: Hover over the dildo and tell him how much you want it. Spread your labia or touch yourself. Slowly lower yourself onto the dildo, savoring every inch. Begin by establishing a slow up-and-down rhythm. This is all about you, girl, so bask in the spotlight as you ride that dildo. Place your hands on either side of his body or against his chest to give you some leverage. He can also hold your arms while you move or you can press them against the bed's headboard. Remember, this is not a position that's comfortable for everyone, and you definitely get a quad workout!

Strap-on Harnesses for Women

Every single day that I worked at Babeland, at least one male/female couple came in to buy a strap-on for her to use on him. And that was ten years ago! These days, women strapping it on to penetrate their partners is more and more popular, and I get dozens of letters every day from couples who have embraced this activity. So what is all the fuss about? Strap-on sex can be exciting, boundary pushing, and extremely intimate for many couples. For men who already enjoy anal penetration, strap-on anal play is another way for your partner to be able to give you what you crave. Plenty of guys just love the way it feels to have a toy that's connected to their partner's body thrusting in and out of them. Some men fantasize about being on the receiving end of a dick for a change, while others like to incorporate strap-on sex into dominant/submissive role-play. For women, strap-on sex is a new way to give their partners pleasure. The harness frees up your hands for other kinds of stimulation and gives you a unique chance to put your whole body behind the anal penetration. It puts you in the driver's seat for a change. Some women get off on being able to give it to their guys, while others experience physical pleasure with the help of some ingenious toys designed especially for strap-on sex.

Your Guide to Choosing a Harness

You can find some strap-on dildos and harnesses sold together in kits, but the best strap-on is the one you "build" yourself by choosing the dildo and the harness. Just like with dildos, when choosing a harness, you have several things to consider. Harnesses can be made of leather, vinyl, nylon, rubber, and different kinds of fabric. They come in a variety of styles and can be basic, embellished, no-nonsense, or glamorous. You can embrace a fetish look with leather and metal hardware, go for a red sparkly superhero harness, or even have a clear plastic see-through harness. The material you choose depends on how you want your harness to look and how much money you want to spend.

Tristan's Harness Picks

Best value harness:
Aslan Pleasure Principle
Harness ($48)

Best see-through harness:
Sportsheets Peek-a-Boo Clear
Harness ($30)

Most stylish harness:
Aslan Prince Vinyl Harness ($85)

Best leather harness:
Stormy Leather Terra Firma
Harness ($65)

Best girly harness:
Outlaw Leather Annie-O
Harness ($115)

In addition to aesthetics, harnesses come in two main styles: one strap and two strap. A one-strap harness has a strap that goes around your hips, one that goes between your legs, and a panel in front (sometimes with a cock ring) where the dildo slips through a hole. Because it fits like a G-string, the center strap rubs against your genitals, which may feel stimulating to some and annoying to others. This style harness tends to fit especially petite women the best.

A two-strap harness has a strap that goes around your hips and two straps that go around your ass cheeks; it fits like a jock strap, leaving your vagina and ass easily accessible and free to be stimulated. It has a panel of material with a hole and a cock ring for the dildo. Some two-strap models have just a cock ring without a panel of material; some styles have a detachable cock ring that can be changed to accommodate different-sized dildos. These are especially good if the dildo you are using is significantly smaller or larger than average. Others have a cock ring that sits on top of the material, so the dildo does not go directly against your body. Some people find that the two-strap harness tends to give them more control than the one-strap model;

the dildo moves around less and is easier to guide. Harnesses have three different types of fasteners: metal D-rings that the material slides through, plastic fasteners similar to straps on a backpack, or metal buckles like on a belt.

You want to choose a harness that fits you well—the snugger and more secure, the better. If you are a larger woman, ask the store for harnesses designed for large women or see whether you can order extra-long straps. I recommend that you try a few different styles on before you buy them; most reputable stores will let you try it on over your clothes. If you order from a catalog or website, see what the return policy is. The majority of dildos will fit in a standard harness, as long as there is a flared base and the dildo isn't excessively large.

Vixen Mistress Dildo and
Annie-O Harness

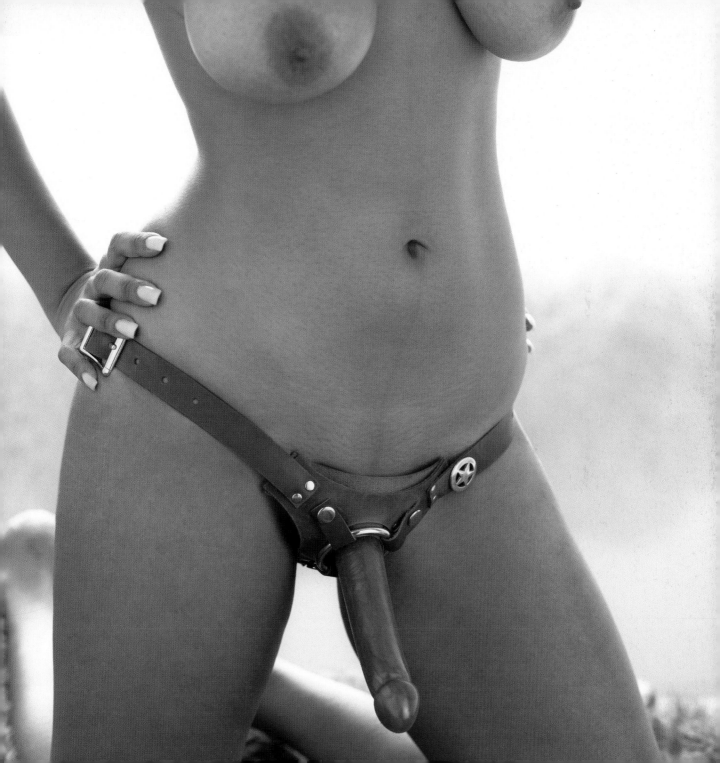

Using a Strap-on Harness

To put on a harness, first buckle all the straps together but keep it loose, slip the dildo through the O-ring, and step into the harness as if it were a pair of underwear or shorts. Then position the dildo, adjust the straps, and tighten them. Or you can put the strap around your hips, put the dildo through the O-ring, then buckle or fasten the other strap (or straps). Make sure you buckle or fasten it so that it's tight against your body; a common mistake beginners make is that they leave it too loose. You want to position the dildo where it's most comfortable for you. Most people like it to sit against the pubic mound so that the bottom of the dildo base rests against the clitoral hood and top of the vulva. If the dildo has a very exaggerated curve, make sure the curve is always aimed toward the front of his body for prostate stimulation (or hers for G-spot stimulation).

Penetrating someone while wearing a strap-on is a learned skill, so give yourself some time to get the hang of it. As a woman doing the penetration, you should experiment with different positions. I know that the first few times I did it, I had my partner in Doggie Style position for several reasons. Doggie Style gives you a clear view of the anus, so you can see what the hell you're doing. The position allows for a good angle of penetration, toward the prostate in men. It's an easy angle to get your balance, establish a rhythm, and get some good thrusting going. So, you may want to start out that way, but you can also try Missionary (usually with legs over the shoulders) or Cowboy (him on top).

Learning how to skillfully wield a strap-on takes practice and patience. If you feel like the dildo is moving around too much or doesn't feel secure, then your harness isn't tight enough and you should adjust it. In the beginning, you may want to guide the dildo with your hand, which will give you more control of exactly where it's going. When your partner is ready for penetration, be gentle and go slowly. Press the tip of the well-lubricated dildo against his opening, and have him come back on it. This may help him feel less vulnerable, and will reassure you that you're not hurting him. Once you are inside him, and he's ready for some movement, begin slowly. You want to establish a thrusting motion with your hips, one that feels good to him and won't tire you out too quickly.

Women can enjoy penetrating men on many different levels. The trust and intimacy between partners can feel especially heightened and very arousing. The naughty, taboo aspects of both anal sex and a woman with a dick can really get her motor going. The power she feels as the penetrating partner can also add to her fantasy and pleasure. Women, you'll be happy to know that strap-on anal sex also has the potential to be physically stimulating for you. There are many different ways for a woman to get pleasure during strap-on sex. For some women, when the base of the dildo rubs against the clitoris and vagina, there is enough friction there to feel fantastic. Some women get enough clitoral stimulation from this action to have an orgasm.

If you want to add a vibrator to the equation, you've got several options. You can try to don a wearable vibrator beneath the harness, but this may be awkward and interfere with the snugness of the harness. A better idea is to use the Buzz Me harness, made by Stormy Leather and equipped with a pocket for a small vibrating egg or a mini vibrator. There are also dildos with hollowed-out bases made for vibrating mini bullets. For double penetration (one for you, one for your partner), you can buy a double dildo made especially for harness use. You want one that is made for use in a harness, not one of those extra-long dongs with two heads. I recommend the Nexus by Vixen: a two-dildos-in-one package designed so the harness wearer can have a dildo inside her vagina while simultaneously penetrating her partner with the other end.

Not Just for Girls: Strap-on Harnesses for Men

When most people think of strap-ons, they picture women wearing them to penetrate either male or female partners. But strap-ons aren't just for girls! Plenty of men use strap-ons, too. Some may have erectile dysfunction or difficulty. Some may like to have a backup for when their penis runs out of steam but their partner doesn't. And some are just looking for a whole new way to have sex!

There is only one harness made especially for men, the Men's Dildo Harness by Canadian company Aslan Leather ($130). On this leather harness, below the opening for the dildo, is a pouch for the man to store his goods. The strap starts behind the pouch, making this more comfortable than a traditional one-strap model that could rub uncomfortably against his genitals. Men can also wear some of the two-strap harnesses previously described. Ask for recommendations from a salesperson or try some on over your underwear to find one that's comfortable. All the advice about choosing a harness and using one in this chapter applies to men as well.

Perfect Pairing: Nexus Double Dildo + Doggie Style Position

Doggie Style is a great position for women who are just starting to explore how to properly wield a new toy between their legs! It gives you a chance to find your center of gravity, practice your hip action, and get used to the rhythm of thrusting. If you like to look at, squeeze, or spank your partner's butt, this gives you the best view and the most access. If couples want to explore dominant/submissive role-play during anal sex, Doggie Style can work well to help you channel your inner mistress and have your partner surrender to your will. If he puts his head down while his butt is in the air, his body is angled well for you to stimulate his prostate. The Nexus ($78 to $120) is an amazing toy because it allows the wearer to be penetrated as she penetrates her partner.

Wearing the Nexus takes a little practice. First, with all the straps loosely fastened, step into the harness. Slide the Nexus into the harness so that the shorter end—which is the one intended for you—is facing your body and the longer end is protruding from the front of the harness. Then, lube up your end and slide it into your vagina. When it feels comfortable, adjust the other end of the dildo and then tighten all the straps on the harness. Now you're ready for action!

I'm assuming you've read the previous chapter all about anal penetration and warm-up, so when you break out the Nexus, his ass has been properly prepared. Lube the other end of the dildo and rub it against his anal opening. Have him take the lead and actually come back onto the dildo; this way, he can control the speed and depth of penetration as well as the angle. Reach around to stimulate his penis and balls; have him continue to come back onto the dildo and show you the speed and rhythm he likes. Then you can take over the thrusting. Hold on to his hips to give yourself more leverage. Run your fingers up and down his back—for a more intense sensation, use your nails!

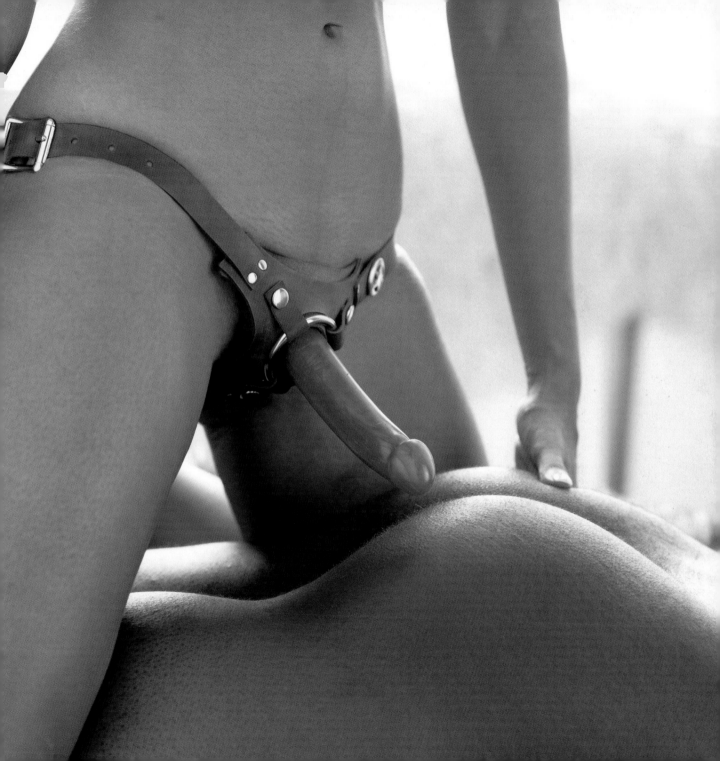

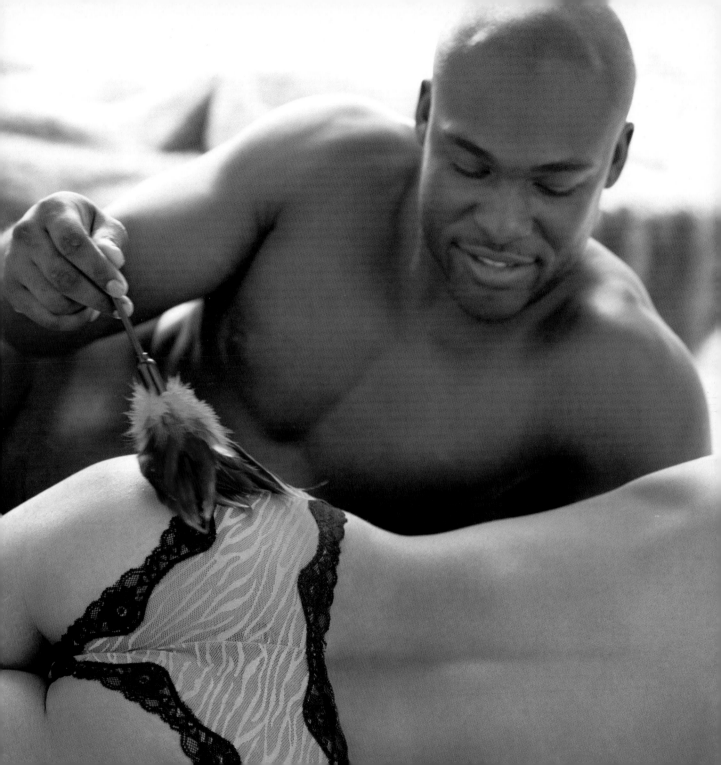

CHAPTER 17

IGNITE YOUR SENSES WITH SENSATION PRODUCTS AND TOYS

If you're looking to have a truly sensual experience when you have sex, one that goes beyond just your genitals, why not stimulate all your senses? Whether it's sight, smell, sound, touch, or taste, the products and toys in this chapter awaken, arouse, and stimulate one or more of your senses. Not only can this add a new component to your lovemaking, but it will also help you and your partner connect with your senses and your whole body. You can use these treats as the first course in an evening-long feast, a surprise addition to shake up a familiar routine, or something fun to inspire playfulness and fantasy.

Feathers: Sensual, Luxurious, Ticklish

There's a reason why in the popular French maid fantasy the maid is usually always carrying a feather duster, and it doesn't have anything to do with cleaning the house! Feathers are sensual, luxurious tools that feel great against the skin and stimulate our touch receptors. They can stroke, flutter, tickle, and tease the flesh. They are a fun way to get someone in the mood without intimidating him or her, so they are a good bet for beginners and lovers who aren't ready for whips and chains. If you want to shake things up in bed but aren't sure how your partner might react to a sensual toy, try a feather toy. It's sure to be fun without being too far out there. You can buy a large single feather (such as a giant ostrich feather) or a feather tickler made of many feathers attached to a handle (similar to a duster). Run a feather tickler down the entire length of your partner's body. Brush the feathers lightly against the skin, then follow each swipe with a kiss. If you're feeling playful, you can use your feather to torture him as you target his ticklish spots. If tickling turns both of you on, check out a wonderful book on the subject, *Erotic Tickling* by Michael Moran, for more information.

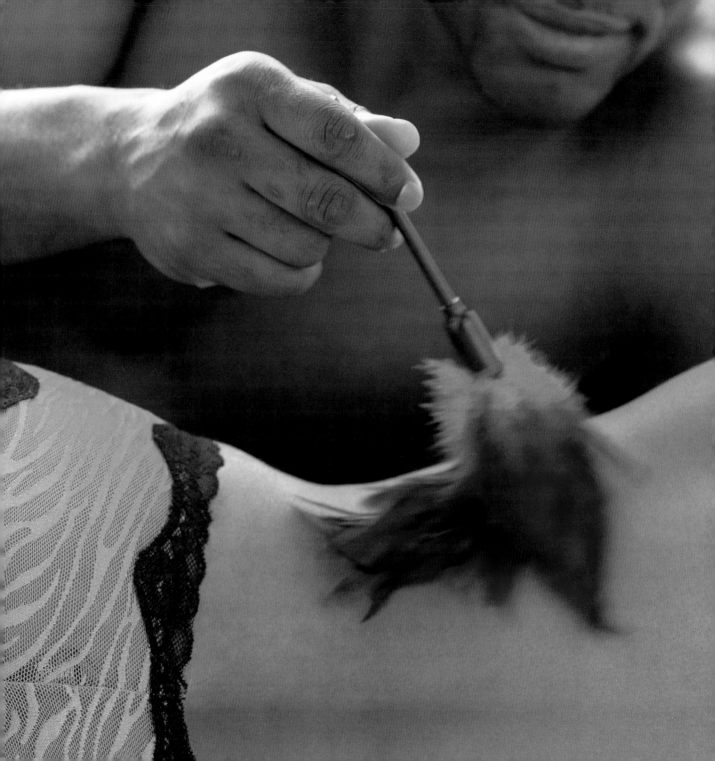

Feathers: Lover's Feather Ticklers by Pipedream ($5)

Massage oil: Babeland Massage Oil in Lavender Vanilla ($13)

Massage oil candle: Jimmyjane Afterglow Candle ($25)

Stimulating gel: O'My Clitoral Pleasure Gel ($20)

Body paint: Shunga Chocolate Body Paint ($9)

Liquid latex: Deviant Liquid Latex ($18)

Massage Oil: Touch Plus Smell = Sexy Fun

Want to combine both touch and smell into one sensual experience? A sensual massage is a great way to start an evening of sexy fun. You don't need to be a licensed masseuse to give a good massage, you just need to be generous, listen to your partner, and use the healing power of touch. Massage oil is easy to find, and you have lots of brands to choose from; in fact, popular lube companies such as K-Y and Astroglide have gotten into the game and now produce their own massage oils. Other good brands are Kama Sutra, Good Clean Love, Babeland, and Good Vibrations Touch Me. There are also massage bars—a solid bar that dissolves into oil as you use it on the skin; these are much are easier to travel with and can be less messy than oils. To add some taste to your indulgent experience, choose a lickable or edible massage oil, which you can rub all over your partner's body, then have fun tracing those spots with your tongue and licking it up.

The most important thing to keep in mind with massage oil is that if does in fact contain oil, it can stain sheets, fabric, and clothes and may be hard to clean up, so make sure you put a towel down first. Oil-based products should not get near your genitals if you're planning to have sex. Oil-based products are bad for vaginas and can cause vaginal infections. Some couples enjoy using silicone lube as a massage oil because it's slick, moisturizing, and, most important, not oil-based; this way, you can transition from massage to sex play without having to switch to a different product.

Massage Oil Candles: Wax Play, without Pain

Candles are a wonderful way to set a romantic mood, and many couples light them to create some sexy ambience in the bedroom. Some folks fantasize about another use for those candles: They want to seductively drip hot wax all over their partner's body, or have it drizzled on them. It looks great in the movies, but the reality doesn't always live up to the hype: If you use the wrong kind of candle, the wax can actually burn someone's skin. If it burns at the correct temperature, you're still left with a lot of cooled wax to clean up. Massage oil candles not only address and fix these common issues, but they also combine two activities in one product. They burn at a very low

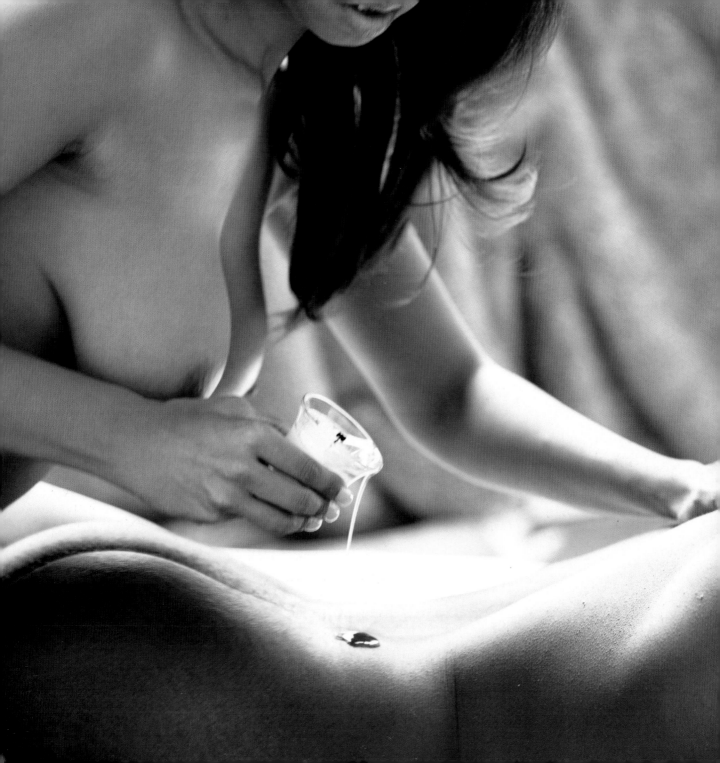

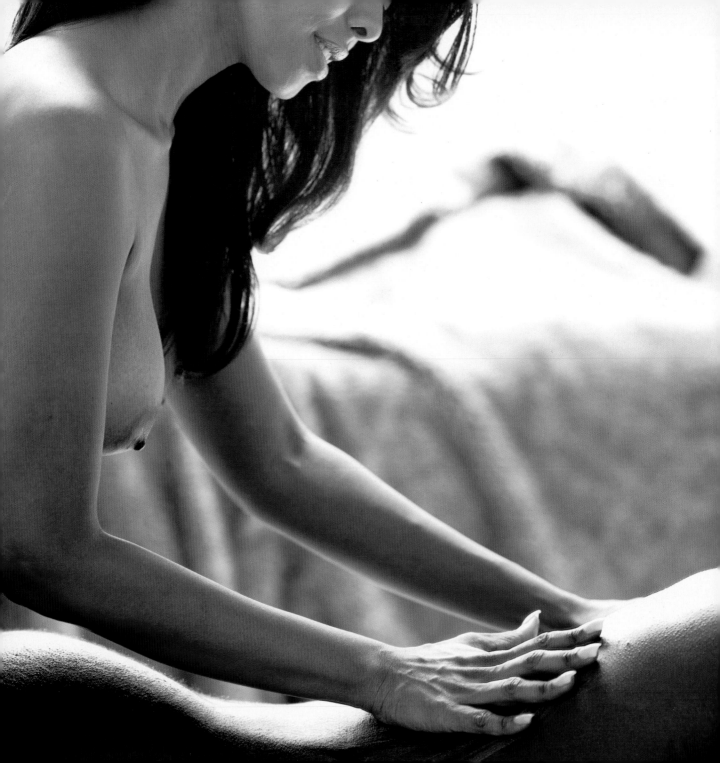

temperature, making it gentle and safe to use without fear of hurting your partner by scorching his skin. Light the candle and let the wax begin to melt. Lift your hand up and away from your partner's body (the farther away the candle, the cooler the wax will be when it hits the skin). Once you've drizzled your partner's body with warm wax, start rubbing your fingers into it and it will transform into silky smooth massage oil. Now, you're ready to give an erotic massage!

Gels and Creams Stimulate Your Sensitive Spots

We all know that the genitals are very sensitive, but some folks like to make them even more sensitive. Stimulating gels and creams such as Rocket Balm, Flower Balm, and Please Pleasure Cream do just that. I recommend the products that contain some kind of natural stimulant, such as menthol or peppermint, over those with chemical stimulants or numbing agents. Stimulating gels and creams created for men stimulate the head and frenulum of the penis; apply a small amount and in a few seconds the area will start to tingle. Those made for women can be used on the clitoris and are formulated to boost the arousal process and make her more sensitive. When you put a tiny bit on the hood or the underside of the clitoris, the area tingles, blood rushes to the genitals, and the entire vulva gets swollen and aroused. I don't recommend you put them on other parts of the labia, and they should definitely not be used internally. You can also use them on men or women's nipples for extra sensation.

Body Paint and Dust: An Edible Treat

If you love the idea of licking chocolate sauce, whipped cream, honey, and other goodies off your partner's body, then you'll love edible body paint and dust. They're just as tasty, but safe for the body, moisturizing to the skin, and easy to clean up afterward. Edible body paints come in different colors and flavors and offer all sorts of fun opportunities. Create a colorful masterpiece on your naked body. Draw a bikini on and have him take it off. Write naughty words on your body and ask your partner to lick them off. Paint your partner's sensitive spots, then erase them with your mouth. Imagine soft baby powder sprinkled on your skin, then nibbled off by someone you love. You can experience that sensation with edible body dust. Some dusts come with a feather, so you can combine the sensuality of feathers against skin with a delicious powder.

Liquid Latex for Temporary Rubber Creations

Rubber can be very, very sexy. Imagine rubber tight against your skin, coating each inch and curve of your body as if you were poured into it. Or it was poured on you. As latex clothing has moved beyond the underground fetish world and into the mainstream, more people have become interested in what it's like to wear rubber bras, dresses, tops, shorts, and other items. Liquid latex is a blend of skin-safe latex that you can pour or brush on the body; it dries in about 10 or 15 minutes, and as it does, it shrinks, becoming tighter against the skin. You can make your own custom, temporary rubberwear out of liquid latex, and it can last for several hours. For some, it's not about fashion at all; they just love the sensation of having liquid latex put on their body, the thrill of watching it dry, and the excitement of having a partner peel it off slowly.

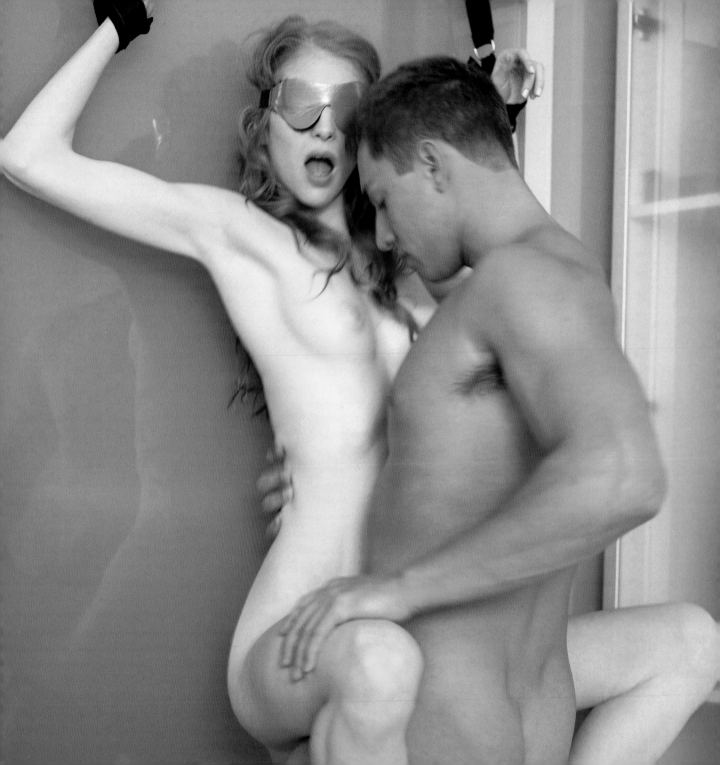

CHAPTER 18

TIE HER UP,
TIE HIM DOWN:

Bondage for Every Budget

When many people recall their first experience of bondage, it usually reaches all the way back to childhood. As part of cops and robbers, cowboys and Indians, or another kids' game, someone had to be restrained at some point. You'd grab a necktie or a belt or something from one of your parent's closets and tie up the bad guys. Some people look back on those experiences as fun memories. Bondage enthusiasts usually remember the first time they were tied up (or tied someone else up) with a lot more detail and glee.

For grown-ups, bondage is an erotic activity with endless possibilities. It seems to transcend categories: Self-described kinky and nonkinky folks alike incorporate different types of bondage into their sex play. If you've ever held down your lover's hands while you were having sex or pinned a partner down to the bed with your body, then you've practiced a form of bondage. That's one of the bonuses of bondage: You can do it without any fancy equipment and you can use what's nearby: a silk scarf, a pair of suspenders, pantyhose—heck, I've used a rolled-up sheet in a pinch. Of course, you can also invest in some great bondage toys and accessories, from the simple to the elaborate.

Bondage is incredibly versatile and can cover lots of erotic territory, from teasing to torment, and everything in between. It's an ideal vehicle to explore explicit power dynamics, because restraining someone embodies dominance, control, power, and authority. And being restrained is a way to submit, surrender, and give oneself over to another.

Your Guide to Playing Safe

Before you begin playing with any bondage toy, you need to sit down with your partner and talk about what you're going to do. Bondage requires a great deal of trust and communication between partners. Share any fears you may have as well as any fantasies. Talk about what the limits are. Are you interested in wearing cuffs, but only on your wrists? Maybe you want to be tied down to the bed. Perhaps you're interested in playing master/slave. Or you want to experiment with a new bondage kit you bought, except you don't want to be blindfolded. If you wear a collar, would you also like him to put you on a leash? If she ties you up and puts on a blindfold, how will you let her know if you want to stop? You should both agree on a safeword: a word that either partner can say to have your bondage play stop, if necessary. Some couples play with two safewords; for example, they use yellow to say "slow down, not so hard, ease up" and red to say "stop." Whatever word you agree on, remember that you can use it at any time.

There are lots of different types of bondage toys, and this chapter will cover some of the most common, including blindfolds, collars, bondage tape, wrist and ankle cuffs, and bondage kits and systems. Except for blindfolds, what these all have in common is that they restrain or bind a part of the body. Whether it's Velcro, a buckle, or a knot, you should always make sure whatever you put someone in is safe. Cuffs and collars should fit well, but not be too tight. You should be able to put two fingers between the item and the person's skin. You never want bondage to put too much strain on parts of the body; the person won't be able to be in that bondage for very long. Better to make your captive more comfortable, so she or he can stay tied up for as long as you want! You should also check in periodically with your partner to make sure that everything still feels okay. If the person in bondage feels pain, tingling, or numbness, take the restraint off immediately.

Blindfolds Can Heighten Your Other Senses

When you take away someone's sense of sight, his other senses become heightened: Noises sound louder, smells are more intense, and even the lightest touch can send chills down the spine. Blindfolds can also help put someone in a particular frame of mind; people wearing them often feel curious and excited as they anticipate what might come next. A blindfold can help someone focus on what's happening to her body, making every sensation stronger.

An effective blindfold is one that someone can't see out of, which may mean it's time to invest in something a little better than that silky sleep mask by the bed (although, to be fair, some sleep masks work amazingly well as blindfolds). Blindfolds come in polyester, satin, leather, and other fabrics, and it's really a matter of personal taste. Some have an elastic strap; others fasten with Velcro or a buckle. Elastic straps usually aren't adjustable, so make sure the blindfold fits well and is not too tight. If you're going to be lying on your back most of the time, then you may not want a blindfold with a buckle, because it can become uncomfortable against the back of your head pretty quickly. Blindfolds should be snug, but not too tight. People who wear contact lenses and a blindfold for a long period of time may find that their lenses dry out or become uncomfortable; keep lens drops handy or have your partner take his lenses out before you begin. When a blindfold comes off, the person will usually be disoriented and extra sensitive to light, so give him some time to readjust to being able to see again.

Collars: Fashion or Fetish

Although they've become more mainstream and some people wear them as a fashion statement, I'm old school when it comes to collars. I say only wear one if someone asks you to. A collar may signify ownership, submission, subservience, surrender, and a whole range of other power dynamics. For many, when a lover puts a collar around her neck, it helps her give up control and become more submissive. Putting a collar on someone is also a great way to

begin a role-playing scene, to transition from your real-life personalities into dominant and submissive, master and slave, or whatever roles you've chosen for the scene. Like other bondage toys, collars can be made of leather, rubber, nylon, and other materials; some collars have Velcro or buckles, and others have a ring where you can insert a lock. For the fashion conscious among you—you know who you are—you can often get a collar to match your wrist and ankle restraints. A collar should be snug around the neck, but never tight, choking, or cutting off circulation; make sure you can fit two fingers between the collar and the person's neck. You can grab the front ring of a collar to pull someone toward you, but never yank someone's collar or drag him by the neck.

Bondage Tape: Easy on, Easy Off

Have you ever seen a movie where someone gets tied up with duct tape? It's quick and easy, and good guys and bad guys alike always seem to have it handy. Sure, duct tape is great for lots of things, but in the real world, bondage is not one

of them. Imagine ripping a Band-Aid off a sensitive part of your body. Now imagine that it's twenty times stickier. Duct tape, and other kinds of tape, are so sticky that after only a minute against someone's skin, they can do serious damage. Luckily, some pervy people have invented an alternative!

Bondage tape is made of a thin plastic, comes in several colors, and is available at most sex toy stores. It comes in a 2-inch (5-cm) -wide roll that looks a lot like packing tape, but this tape isn't sticky, so it's safe for your skin. Bondage tape clings to itself, which is how it stays in place, but it won't stick to hair or skin. I love bondage tape because it's inexpensive and easy to use—you don't even have to tie a knot to tie someone up. However, some practice isn't a bad idea, because ideally you want to keep it as flat against the skin as possible; when it bunches up, it can cause pinching. Wrap it around wrists, arms, thighs, and ankles, make a blindfold, tie someone to a chair. When you're ready to set your captive free, you can unroll it (which takes some patience) and reuse it, or simply cut it off and throw it away.

Cuff 'Em

Wrist and ankle cuffs come in a variety of price ranges and styles and can be made of nylon, vinyl, leather, rubber, or other materials. If they are not made of a soft material, consider getting cuffs that are lined with some cushioning, such as fleece, to make them more comfortable (which means you or your partner can stay in them longer!). Wrap wrist cuffs just above the wrist bone and secure them; they usually have Velcro or buckles. Cuffs should not be too loose, but they should never be tight. You can use wrist cuffs alone, ankle cuffs, or both.

Once the cuffs are on, you have some choices to further restrain your partner. Each cuff has a ring on it to attach things to, and you can use a snap hook (found at hardware stores) or another type of clip to attach the cuffs to each other. You can clip cuffs together over someone's head, in front of her, or behind her. The important thing is that the position you "lock" her arms into isn't putting too much strain on her body. Or you may not want his wrists together, but spread apart, and tethered to something sturdy. This is

especially true of ankles, because most people prefer to have their partner's legs spread for easy access! Slip a long scarf, belt, necktie, or piece of rope through the ring and tie each wrist or ankle to a chair, the slats in your headboard, the bedposts, or something else solid and stable. You have other options as well for restraining someone, which you'll read about in the next section. If you're interested in rope or other types of bondage, see the end of this chapter for some resources.

What about Real Handcuffs?

I'm sorry to burst your cop/criminal fantasy, but you should never use traditional metal handcuffs in your sex play. I still see them in people's bedrooms and they're sold at sex shops, but they really are not safe to use to restrain someone. Most handcuffs do not have a working safety latch to keep them from closing too tightly around the wrist; they can cut off your circulation, cut into your wrists, and do serious damage to someone. Keep the handcuffs around as props, but don't actually use them!

Bondage Kits: Create Your Own Experience

Bondage kits come complete with several different pieces that work together to create a great bondage experience. Some kits make it possible to do bondage in an ordinary bedroom without any fancy equipment; if you don't have a slatted headboard or a four-poster bed, you can transform any ordinary bed into your own bondage playground! Here are some of the best kits available:

- **Sportsheets Under the Bed Restraint System** ($45): This clever kit is perfect for folks who want to be able to tie someone down to the bed, but don't have the type of bed that you can attach anything to. Two long, strong nylon straps go between the mattress and the box spring or around the bed frame, and they can be adjusted to fit any size bed. Lay them vertically and the straps come around the head and foot of the bed, resting at the top and bottom of the mattress, so you can restrain hands and feet there. Lay them horizontally and restrain someone's arms and legs on either side of the bed. At both ends of each strap is a clip that you attach the nylon and Velcro cuffs to (all are included in the kit). Of course, you can use any set of wrist and ankle cuffs with the straps.

- **The Sportsheet Bondage Bed Sheet Set** ($230): Available in queen and king size, the Sportsheet is a velvety mattress cover. It comes with four "anchor pads," thick pads with Velcro that stick to the sheet and stay in place; each pad has a clip on it to which you can attach wrist and ankle cuffs (or you can use your own). Once your sweetie is clipped to the pads, he (or she) isn't going anywhere!

- **Liberator Shapes Black Label** ($115 to $285): You read about Liberator Shapes in the previous chapter, and the same company makes a line of shapes that feature black velvety covers that come equipped with easy-to-use bondage attachments to which you can clip cuffs with a special quick-release clip (also made by Liberator Shapes).

- **Sportsheets Deluxe Door Jam Kit** ($40): Have you ever fantasized about being able to tie up your partner in a standing position, but you're not quite ready to invest in an expensive wooden frame or you can't drill holes for eye hooks into the molding? You can turn any doorway into a bondage device with this inventive kit. Slip these four nylon straps with clips on one end and plastic stoppers on the other over the top of the door and under the bottom. Close the door, and voilà, you've got a sturdy, nonpermanent bondage setup right in your house! These are also great for romantic getaways, because they won't cause any damage to a hotel room.

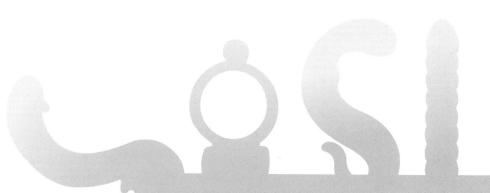

Tristan's Top Picks: Bondage Toys

Best for shy beginners: Sportsheets Vanilla Bondage Kit ($10 to $15)

Most economical bondage: Tickled Pink Restraints ($14)

Best bondage kit: KinkLab Submissive Bondage Kit ($130)

Great for a bed without posts: Sportsheets Under the Bed Restraint System ($45)

Most sexy and stylish: Aslan Leather Jaguar Cuffs ($70)

Splurge purchase: Perforated Bolero Straitjacket at the Stockroom ($465)

The Super Sex Sling

This sling gives you a bondage experience without the work of attaching or
hooking something up to the bed or
doorframe. She can lie back against the
padded neck support while the suspension straps and soft Velcro cuffs hold her
legs in place. Keeping her legs suspended puts her pelvis at the right angle
for him to easily thrust. The straps are
adjustable which allows for maneuver-
ability and position options. The padded
neck support and cuffs minimize tension
on the hips and back, which means you
last longer and have stronger orgasms.

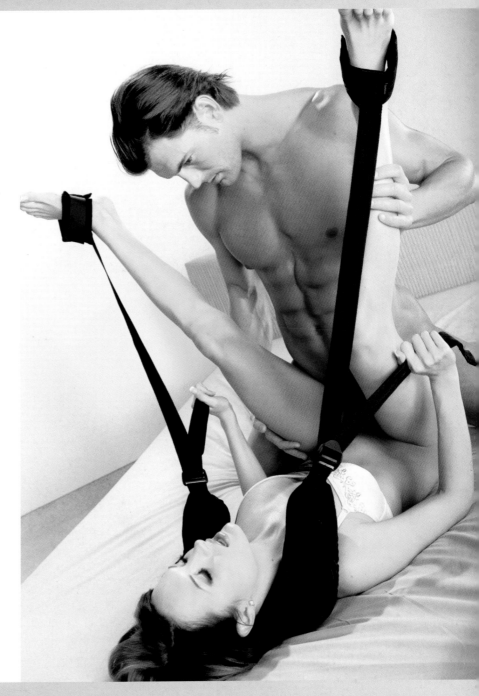

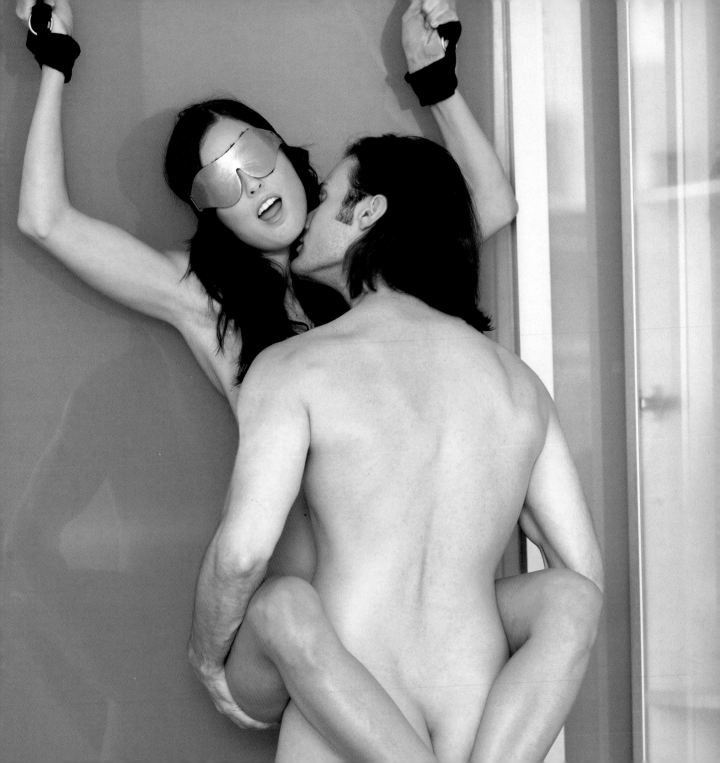

Resources for Advanced Bondage

Books

Bondage for Sex by Chanta Rose

Erotic Bondage Handbook by Jay Wiseman

The Seductive Art of Japanese Bondage by Midori

Shibari You Can Use: Japanese Rope Bondage and Erotic Macramé by Lee Harrington

Two Knotty Boys Showing You the Ropes by Two Knotty Boys

Videos

Midori's Expert Guide to Sensual Bondage (Vivid Ed)

Nina Hartley's Guide to Bondage Sex (Adam & Eve)

Nina Hartley's Guide to Erotic Bondage (Adam & Eve)

Rope Bondage: Precision and Persuasion with Rope (SMTech Educational)

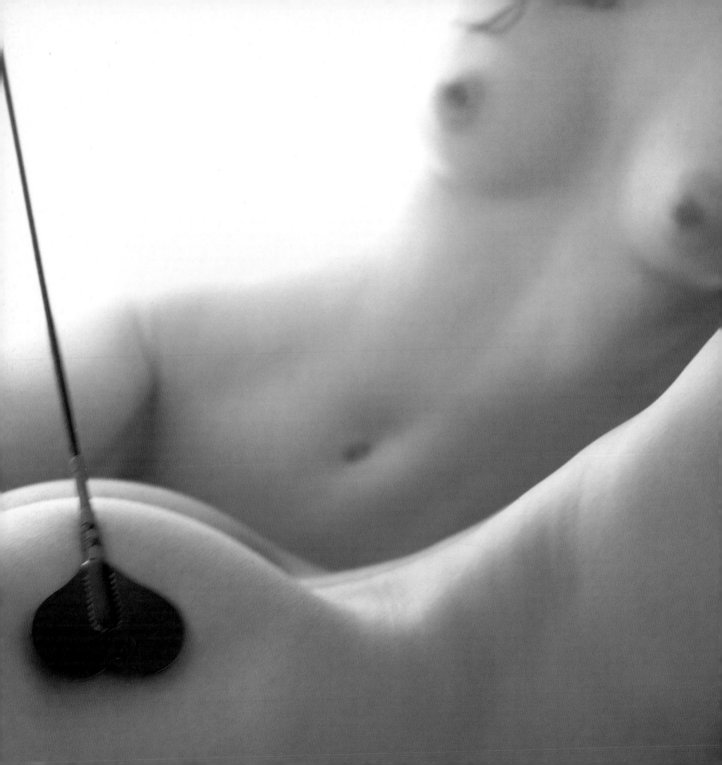

CHAPTER 19

CRACK THE WHIP!

Kinky Toys for Fantasy and Fetish

BDSM is an umbrella term that describes an intimate journey that people take together, where they may explore the boundaries of pain and pleasure, the limits of their own minds and bodies, and even altered states of consciousness.

BDSM stands for three different, yet related, practices:

- Bondage and discipline ("B & D"): constraining someone and punishing him or keeping him in line

- Dominance and submission ("D/S"): creating a dynamic where one partner is dominant—he or she is in charge of the scene—and the other is submissive—he or she submits to the dominant

- Sadism and masochism or sadomasochism (SM): the exploration of different intense physical sensations and/or psychological and emotional states; sadists enjoy inflicting pain, discomfort, or punishment on others, and masochists enjoy receiving it

Most people practice some combination of the three, although certainly some may gravitate toward one more than the others.

In chapter 17, I talked about some different types of sensation play, and most couples who practice BDSM want to take sensation play to another level, giving and/or receiving very intense sensations. These same folks often like to ride the line between pleasure and pain. Sometimes, people who are unfamiliar with BDSM cannot understand how pain can be erotic, pleasurable, and actually desirable. We usually associate pain with physical discomfort and suffering. Sex is supposed to be about feeling good, and what feels good about pain? Well, in actuality, pain can be extremely pleasurable for some people. For one thing, there can be a very fine line separating pleasure and pain, and many people like to explore different sensations that test the borders as well as their endurance, strength, and resilience. Second, when the body experiences pain, it releases endorphins, which are feel-good chemicals that cause you to feel aroused and euphoric, kind of like a

natural high. BDSM play may also have an intense emotional component, where someone has the opportunity through role-playing to test boundaries and explore fantasies and even fears.

Although the previous chapter discussed bondage toys, this chapter covers some of the other toys most commonly used in BDSM play, including nipple clamps, paddles, slappers, crops, and floggers. One important note: Anyone can experiment with these toys. You don't need to join a BDSM club or identify yourself with a BDSM community or lifestyle. But if you're interested in moving beyond experimentation and exploring more advanced activities, I advise you to seek out experienced folks who are into BDSM who can show you the ropes. Local BDSM organizations and stores often sponsor workshops by some of the leading practitioners and teachers in the BDSM community.

Nipple Clamps Offer a Pinch for Pleasure

Chests, breasts, and nipples are all wonderful erogenous zones on our bodies. Both men and women's nipples can be very sensitive, and the level of sensitivity varies from person to person. Lots of folks like their nipples licked, sucked, rolled between fingers, tugged gently, and even pinched. If you love it when your partner plays with your nipples and especially enjoy hard pinching, then you may want to try a pair of nipple clamps. Nipple clamps are small clips attached to a chain, and they come in a wide variety of styles. The best starter set for beginners are tweezer-style or adjustable nipple clamps. Other nipple clamps, as well as other pinching implements (including clothespins, paper clips, or hair clips), are not adjustable at all; their clamping strength might be too intense to start out with for a lot of people. Tweezer-style nipple clamps have a small ring that lets you adjust how much it clamps.

With adjustable clamps, you can start out with the loosest clamping and work your way up to a tighter and more severe pinch. Take your partner's nipple and rub it until it's hard. Place each side of the clamp on the nipple, then slowly begin to

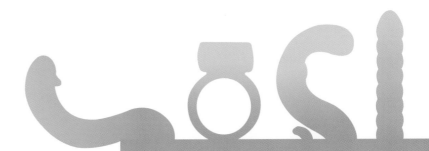

Tristan's Top Picks: BDSM Toys

Nipple clamps: Spartacus Tweezer Clamps ($15 to $20)

Paddle: Stormy Leather Gentle Persuasions Paddle ($60)

Slapper: Stormy Leather Slapper ($33)

Crop: Ruff Doggie Styles Heart Crop ($40)

Flogger with rubber tails: Sportsheets Rubber Whip ($8 to $20)

Flogger with leather tails: Heartwood Deerskin Suede Short Lightweight Flogger ($185)

You're Worth the Splurge: Luxury Crop

If you visit the high-end lingerie shop Agent Provocateur or its website (agentprovocateur.com) and look under whips in the accessories section, you'll find a gorgeous riding crop (yes, they've misnamed a crop a whip, but we'll forgive them). With dazzling Swarovski crystals on the handle and a beautiful leather body, it's one of the best tools for your blinged-out fantasy ($225).

slide the ring toward the nipple to tighten it. Check in with your partner to see what feels good. When you put a clamp on a part of the body, you cut off the circulation to that area. The nipples can get very sensitive, so tugging on the chain between the clamps sends a zing throughout the body. Although it hurts to varying degrees when you put the clamps on and tug at them, it feels a hell of a lot worse when the clamps come off. The blood quickly rushes back to the area in a big burst, and bang, your brain registers pain. So, if your partner is a beginner, leave nipple clamps on for less than a minute before you take them off. You can gradually work your way up to longer amounts of time, but you shouldn't leave clamps on for more than 15 minutes.

Paddles, Slappers, and Crops: Ouch, That's Good

Lots of people get very turned on by spanking. Slapping someone's butt cheeks can be gentle and sensual or deliberate and painful; either way, the consistent smacks release endorphins into the bloodstream and fuel the body's arousal. Although the ass is usually the target of a spanking, you can also slap the thighs and other fleshy parts of the body; always avoid bones and joints, such as the tailbone and the back of the knees. In addition to the physical experience, getting spanked can be punishment for being naughty, a master's order to submit to pain, or part of another role-playing fantasy. Besides your hands, you can smack someone with a paddle, a slapper, or a crop. Most of them can produce a light sensation or a heavy, painful one depending on how much force is behind it.

Most paddles have a broad round or oval striking part and a short handle. Paddles are made of leather, vinyl, rubber, wood, acrylic, and other materials—generally, the harder the material, the more intense the sensation it can produce. They come in a variety of colors, and some feature stars, hearts, or other shapes on them.

Slappers tend to be longer, rectangular, and have a more narrow spanking area. A slapper can be made of one single piece of leather, one piece cut into several strips, or two pieces of leather sewn together at one end. Slappers with multiple pieces of leather tend to make a much louder noise than paddles, so they

can be as much a sensory head trip as a physical one. In general, slappers can produce a harder slap or a stingier one compared to a paddle, which has a larger surface area to diffuse the impact.

Crops are long rods with a small flat loop or a solid piece of leather on the end. The end piece is the part you slap with, which means crops have the smallest slapping area of the three.

Before you introduce your sweetheart to it, it's a good idea for you to try out a paddle, slapper, or crop on a fleshy part of your own body to get an idea of what your partner is going to feel. The key to a good spanking with a paddle, slapper, or crop is to start slowly, warm up the butt, and not rush to spank too hard. Begin with very light flicks, and alternate each one with a nice rub of your hand. You want to gradually build up to firmer swats. Talk to your partner, pay attention to body language, and pace the spanking accordingly. One of my favorite spanking toys—which is especially good for beginners—is a paddle that's smooth leather on one side and soft faux fur on the other. You can alternate each strike with a soothing rub of the sensual fur.

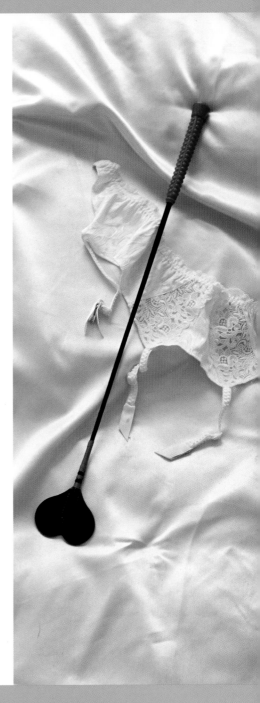

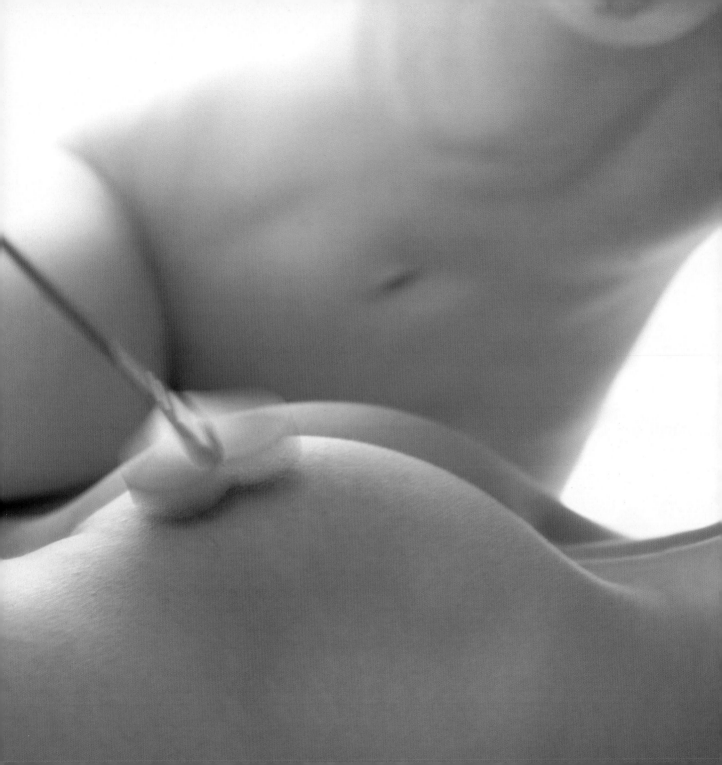

Floggers: From Fantasy to Real Deal

Floggers—sometimes called cat-o'-nine-tails or simply whips—have a handle and multiple "tails"—strips of material that are the same length and width. The handle can be made of leather, plastic, wood, or another material, and the tails are usually made of leather or rubber. There are two kinds of floggers: inexpensive, light floggers (sometimes called fantasy floggers) found in many sex toy stores and expensive, handcrafted floggers geared for the serious BDSM player and sold in leather and fetish stores.

Flogging can produce a range of sensation from light smacks to heavy thuds, depending on the type of flogger and the power behind the strike. Some people enjoy the different sensations a flogger can produce: Slaps, stings, and thuds can feel good and release endorphins.

Fantasy floggers are good for beginners or those interested in exploring light flogging as part of fantasy role-playing. If you're looking for a starter flogger, I recommend one that is relatively short, because it's easier to control. If you want leather, make sure the tails are made of a soft leather, such as deerskin or suede. Sportsheets also makes floggers with very thin, stretchy pieces of rubber, which are good for novices.

To use a flogger you want to hold the handle and aim the ends of the tails at your target. You can swing the flogger over your shoulder, then forward to the person's body, or you can swing it sideways. You should flog only the fleshy parts of the body, such as the butt cheeks, thighs, and upper back; always avoid joints, bones, the spine, the lower back (because of the kidneys), the neck, and the face. Just like with spanking, you want to start gently and work your way up to more intensity.

BDSM Resources

The Ultimate Guide to Sexual Fantasy
by Violet Blue

The Toybag Guide to Clips and Clamps by Jack Rinella

Naughty Spanking Stories from A to Z edited by Rachel Kramer Bussel

Screw the Roses, Send Me the Thorns: The Romance and Sexual Sorcery of Sadomasochism by Philip Miller and Molly Devon

The New Bottoming Book by Janet W. Hardy and Dossie Easton

The New Topping Book by Dossie Easton and Janet W. Hardy

Flogging by Joseph W. Bean

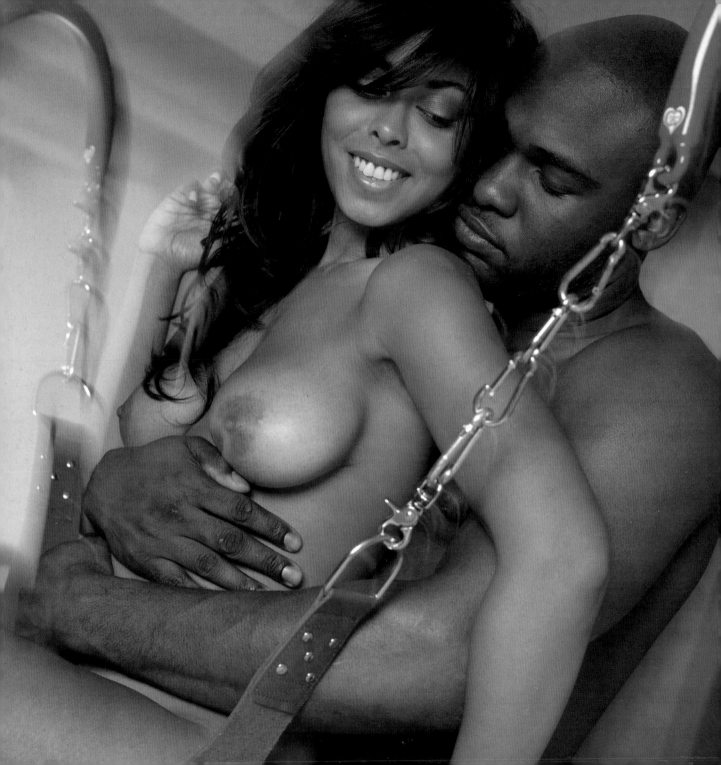

CHAPTER 20

GROWN-UP SWING SETS:
Bedroom Gear and Sex Furniture

I've talked about lots of toys and products meant to inspire, enhance, and rev up your sex life. For those of you who want to go even further in your consumption of sex stuff, listen up: There is furniture made just for sex. That's right, it's time to leave the comfort of your bed for the excitement of creative shapes, sex swings, slings, and other contraptions.

Get a Little Lift with Sex Swings

Sex swings are swings that look similar to hammocks, but were designed especially for sex play and intercourse. Because they must hold your body weight, they are made to be hung with chain from a weight-bearing beam in the ceiling or used with a freestanding metal frame (which is sold separately). If you find sex in the bed has gotten boring, if you're looking for a dramatic way to make over your bedroom environment, or if the idea of having sex while being suspended in the air appeals to you, then you may want to invest in a sex swing ($120 to $500).

There are several different swings on the market. They are usually made of nylon and resemble a hammock, one solid piece with about a dozen adjustable straps on all sides; some are simply a series of wide, padded straps that are connected to each other. Some have a support bar at the top and bottom. Each swing is slightly different, but they all operate on the same concept: to suspend one or both partners in the air for sex. The Bungee Sexperience ($380) takes the concept of a sex swing and combines it with the bouncing motion of a bungee cord.

There are many different positions you can get into in sex swings. One is where the woman sits or lies back in the swing and the man stands in front of her. For women who enjoy being on their backs during sex but don't like their partner's weight on them, the Love Swing makes a face-to-face, him-on-top position possible. She can turn over and you can experiment with different variations of Doggie Style. If you've tried sitting positions and like them, but find they put too much strain on your body, the swing is a good alternative, especially for people with bad backs; you can both sit in a swing for Cowgirl and Reverse Cowgirl. Because the swing totally supports one or both partners' bodies, you feel almost weightless in it. Partners can touch each other's bodies, make eye contact, and communicate.

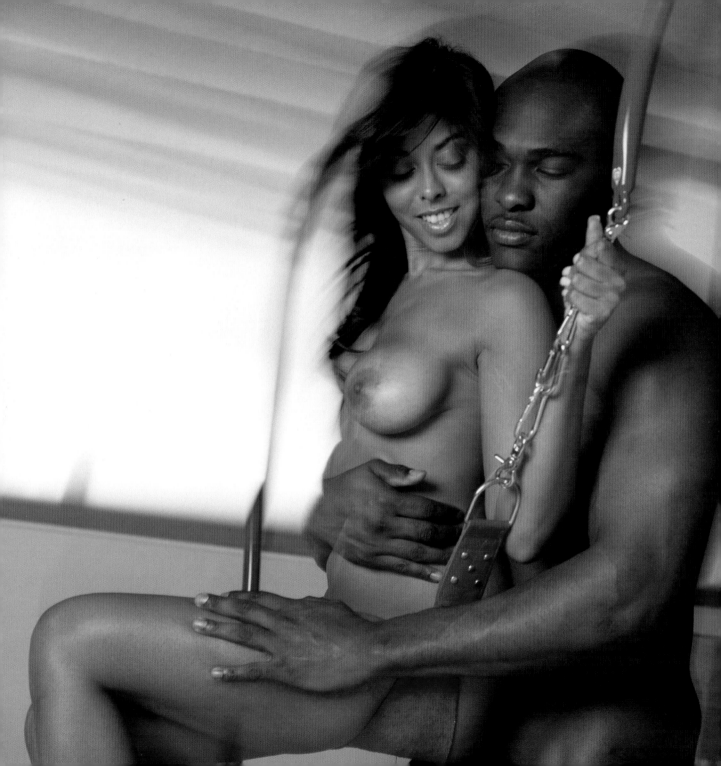

Get into Compromising Positions with Sex Slings

Slings ($400 to $600) are a staple at BDSM and fetish parties and clubs. Slings are not that much different in concept from a swing; they, too, are designed to be hung from a ceiling beam or used with a freestanding metal frame. Unlike some swings that are a series of straps, slings are always one continuous piece—made of nylon webbing or leather, either solid or in a basketweave style— and may have leg or other attachments. The difference between a swing and a sling is primarily aesthetic and functional. Slings tend to be sold in leather and BDSM stores and appeal to people of all genders and sexual orientations; they aren't built just for intercourse, and they are used most often with one partner lying back in the sling and the other one standing or sitting. Swings are marketed to couples, can have more adjustable points than a sling, and are designed with intercourse positions in mind.

There are also body slings (also called travel or portable slings), which have the straps of a swing/sling without the suspension ($50 to $200). One type of body sling is a combination of a head and neck support piece and long leg straps with stirrups on the end. This is ideal for Missionary position where she wants to put her legs up on his shoulders; with the body sling, he doesn't have to hold her ankles or legs, so his hands are free to do other things. With another type, you can actually strap your partner to your body for more stability during standing positions. JT's Stockroom makes a beautiful leather travel sling for women ($230) with ankle and thigh cuffs and a padded neckpiece that lets you put your partner's body in very compromising positions without having to set up a sling!

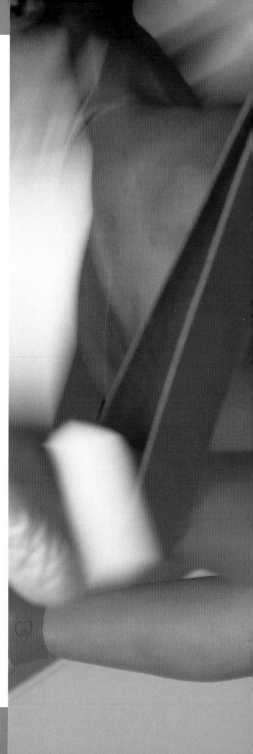

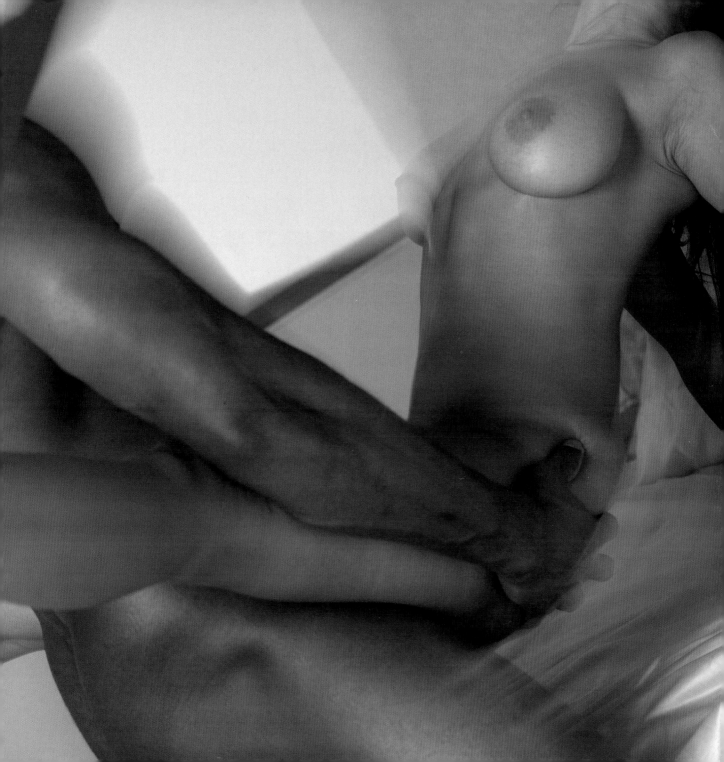

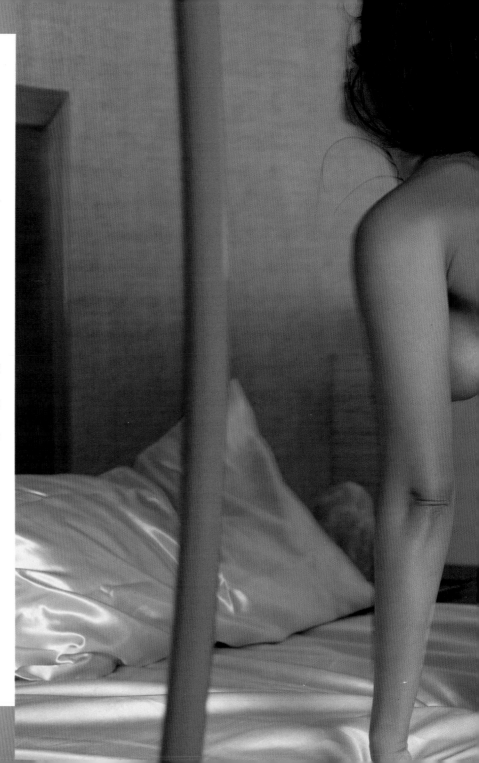

Bonk'er Puts Your Bed to Work

The Bonk'er ($450 to $800), made by a company called Bonkum, is a piece of sex furniture that has elements of both a sling and a frame and you use it with your bed. The Bonk'er works best with beds that have frames up off the ground slightly. It's a metal frame with two curved handles that look like tall, thin candy canes. When assembled, each foot of the frame slides under one side of your bed frame, so that the curved handles stand up alongside the side of the bed curving toward each other. A long, wide piece of leather clips into the holes at either end of the curves; this is the "seat strap." Also clipped to the holes are leg straps that hang down toward the bed. You can use the Bonk'er to hold on to for leverage while you have intercourse and to get into different and unique positions. You can elevate your partner's body, put her legs in the straps and into the air, bend her over the seat strap, then hold onto the handles for more powerful thrusting.

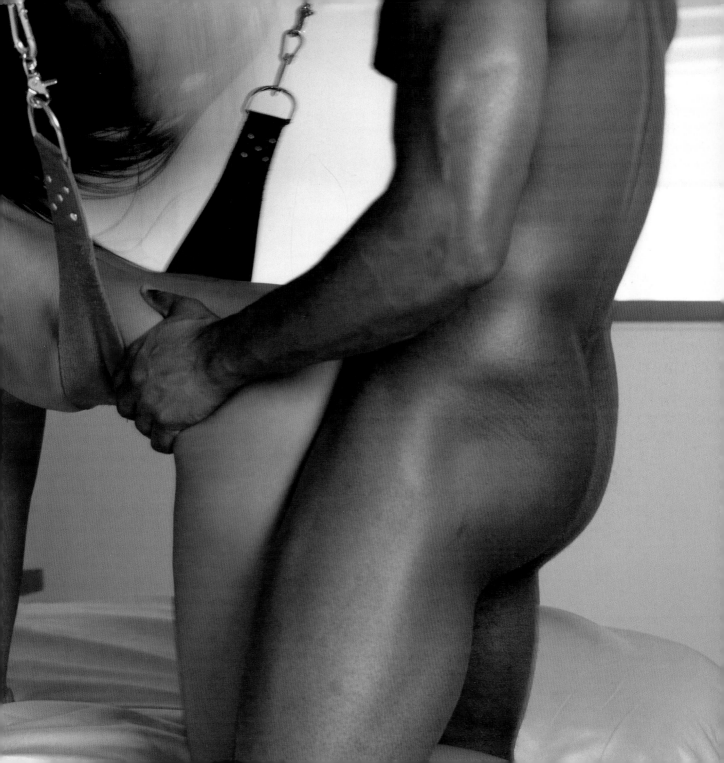

Bedroom Gear and Sex Furniture Websites

Liberator Shapes:
LiberatorShapes.com

Love Swing: LoveSwing.com

Effortless Sex Swing:
JustaSwinging.com

Passion Swing: PassionSwing.com

Sex Swing Store:
SexSwingStore.com

Extreme Restraints Sex Furniture:
ExtremeRestraints.com/sex-furniture_167/

Bonk'er: Bonkum.com

Monkey Rocker: MonkeyRocker.com

Get the Perfect Angle with Liberator Shapes

Liberator Shapes are very unique products that almost no other company has been able to duplicate. They are extra-firm pillows in different shapes that were designed especially for sex. They have soft, velvety covers that are removable, water resistant, and machine washable. The idea behind them is simple: Sex is all about angles, and these shapes help you get the best angle possible. They're also great for people of all sizes and shapes, and those with back pain and other mobility issues. I've personally used all the different shapes and think they are fantastic. Have you ever put a pillow under your butt to give your partner an easier time while he goes down on you? Or do you like to put a pillow underneath your hips in Tailgate position? Pillows tend to sink down and slip, but the small triangular Wedge ($85) gives you the support you need and stays put. The larger triangular Ramp ($140) makes all sorts of positions possible and puts your bodies at a perfect angle for G-spot and P-spot stimulation. There are about a dozen different shapes, including a cube for sitting positions, a half-moon shape that actually rocks, and a large rectangle that pairs nicely with other shapes. Because of the material, you can put shapes together and they'll stay put without slipping.

The same company also makes sex furniture, including Esse ($425 to $450), an S-shaped chair that makes face-to-face positions especially fun; Equus ($375 to $425), a long bench that works great next to the bed; Freestyle ($275), an oversized Ramp with a rounded end; and Zeppelin ($360 to $600), a huge circular piece that looks like a giant beanbag but has a lot more support. For couples who are tired of sex in a bed, but find sex on other furniture in the house challenging, awkward, or uncomfortable, Liberator Shapes are a great way to have new places to do it.

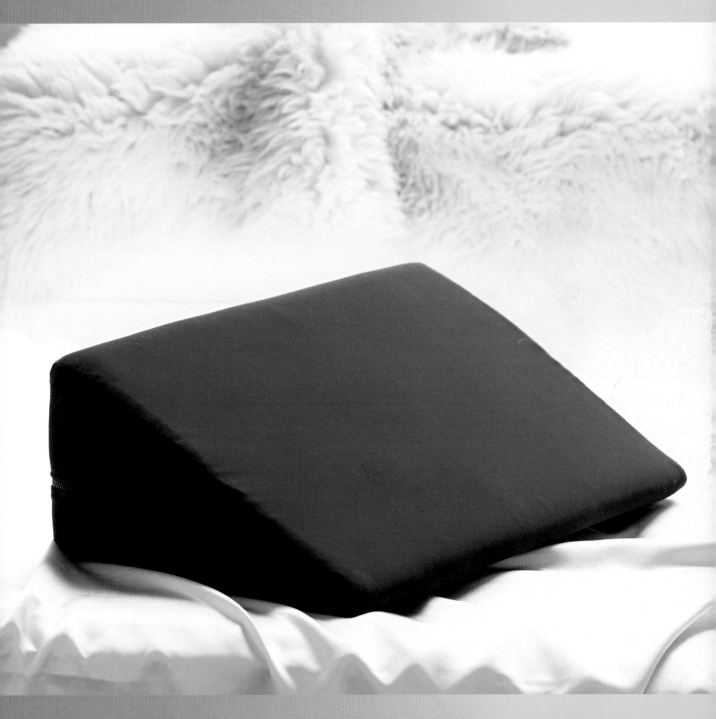

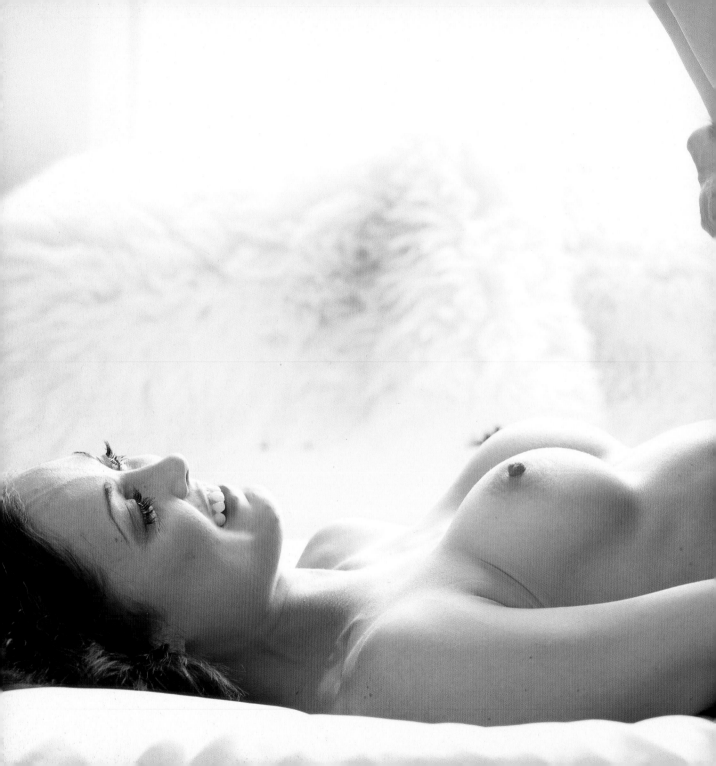

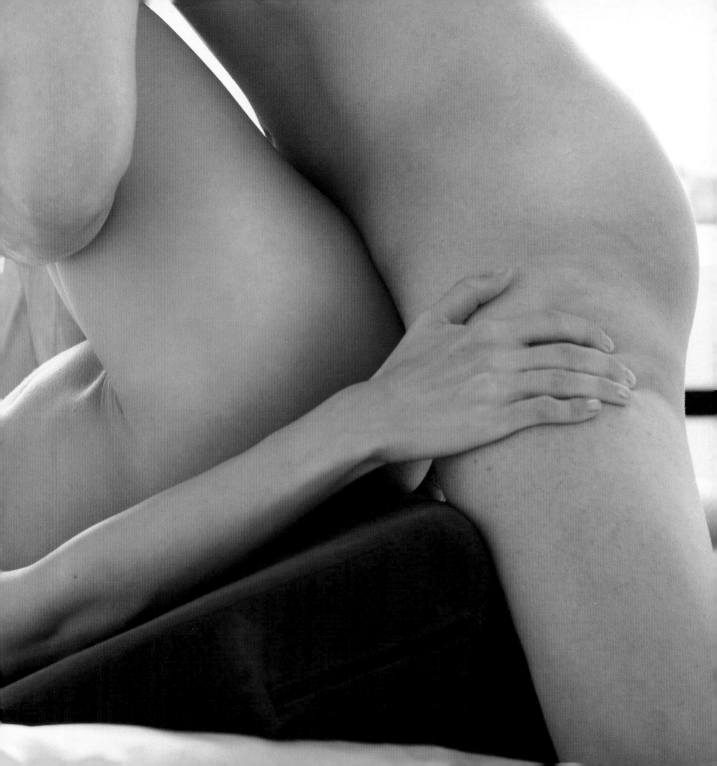

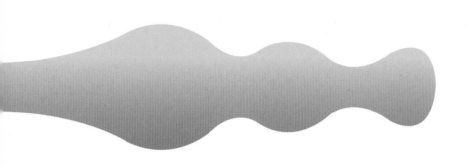

The Bondage Liberator

Esse gives you great support to explore a number of sexual positions. The curved shape supports your head, neck, and back, making it a great option for those who have back issues and need cushioning during vigorous thrusting. Equipped with wrist, thigh, and ankle cuffs and multiple attachments to lock them down, the Esse is a playful way to incorporate light bondage into your sexplay.

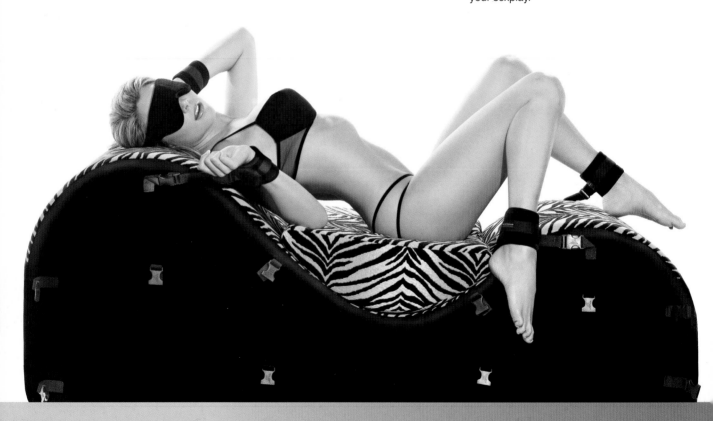

Rock Your Way to Orgasm with the Fetish Fantasy Tilt Master

Sex is about movement, and hitting hot spots like the G-spot, P-spot, and clitoris is about having the right angles. The Fetish Fantasy Tilt Master gives you both the movement and the perfect angles every time. The curved seat allows her to comfortably relax into any position without slipping off. The EZ-grip handles give her support while he thrusts, particularly in positions where her legs are elevated or thrown over his shoulders. The rounded bottom lets you rock your way to an even more incredible orgasm. Best of all, this toy is inflatable so it discreetly tucks away after use and can be easily packed for hot getaways.

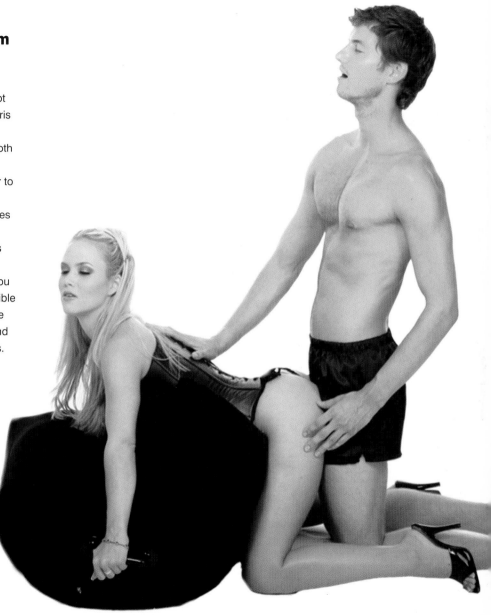

The Liberator Wedge/ Ramp

This combo locks together to give angled support, which is great for G-spot stimulation. This is a great toy for making basic positions like doggie style entry and missionary even hotter with less stress on the back and knees. The angle also gives him an enticing view of your backside, which is a real turn-on.

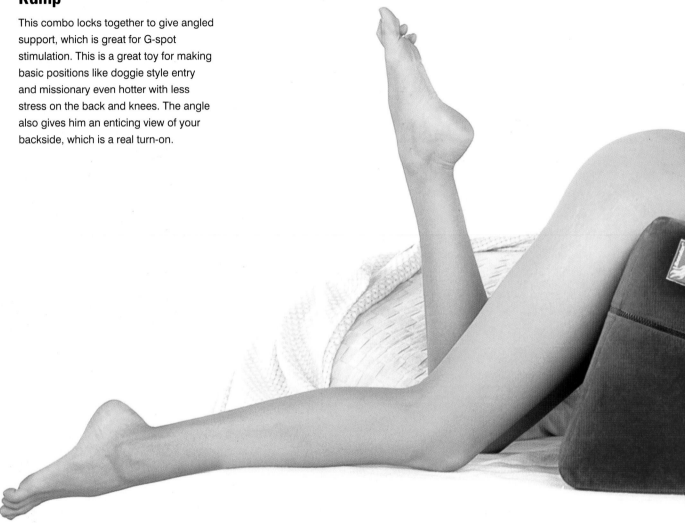

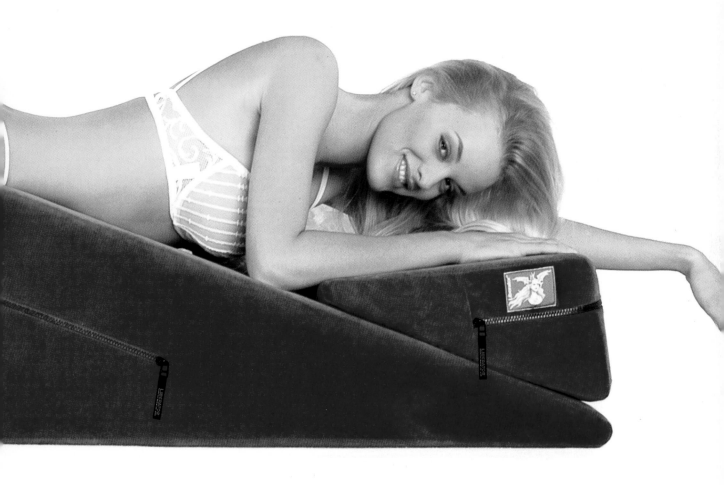

You're Worth the Splurge: Monkey Rocker

The Monkey Rocker ($800 to $950) is the ultimate sex chair for one, and a great masturbation toy for women and men who love penetration. Basically, you sit on the chair, and, as you rock back and forth, a dildo that is attached below moves in and out of you. You can use any harness-compatible dildo you want, because you simply mount it onto the movable arm piece and secure it with an adjustable strap and a cock ring. You control the speed and depth with your motion. You can face either direction, mimicking face-to-face positions or those where your partner enters you from behind.

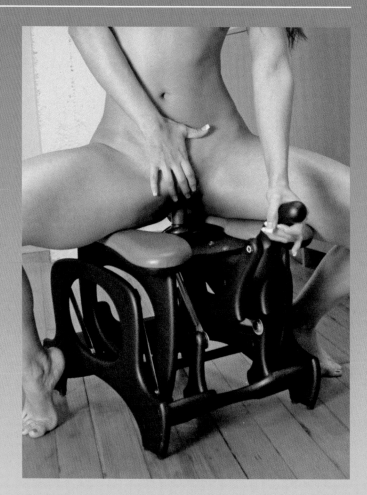

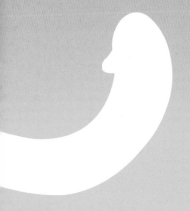

Multiple Orgasms Multiple Ways with the Sybian

The Sybian Sex Machine isn't a new toy but it is one that has gotten a lot of recent attention due to its regular inclusion on *The Howard Stern Show*. Essentially the Sybian is shaped like a small rounded stool that you straddle. The entire area vibrates giving you great clitorial and vulval stimulation. You can attach dildo-like vaginal insert which provides penetration and rotates within the vagina. Combined you have incredible stimulation of the clitoris, G-spot, and the inner and outer vagina. Multiple sensations give an incredible orgasmic experience. As far as sex toys go, it is definitely one of the most sophisticated.

Ride it like a Rock Star

The Star Fuck Machine is perfect for those looking for something a little wild. A round base that comes with different sized dildo attachments it's a great toy for vaginal or anal penetration. Mount the dildo and use the remote control to find your perfect speed and depth of strokes. With eight different settings you can switch it up from slow and easy to deep intense thrusting. The best thing about this toy is that your partner doesn't need to miss out on the fun. The remote control is wireless and can be used from up to 20 feet away so you can turn the reins over to your partner and let them decide how fast or slow to go. You get a great penetration experience and they get to see you take the ride.

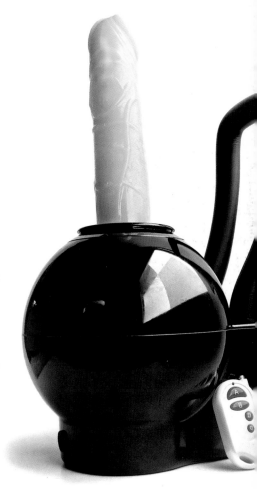

CHAPTER 21

WETTER IS BETTER:

Lubricants to Enhance Your Pleasure

Lube makes everything wetter and therefore better! Lubricants used to only be marketed very discreetly to postmenopausal women, because after menopause, most women experience vaginal dryness. But lube is for people of all genders, sexual orientations, and ages. Like many other elements of the sex toy industry, lube makers finally caught up with consumer needs, and there is now a wide array of lubricants from which to choose.

Although the vagina may produce enough lubrication when a woman is aroused, that's not always the case. Sometimes, you can be very turned on, but the amount of lubrication your body produces doesn't reflect that. How much we lubricate depends on many different factors, including our menstrual cycle, stress, exercise, diet, dehydration, medications (over-the-counter and prescription), and drugs. Arousal and wetness don't always go hand in hand. Sometimes, the vagina does lubricate, but just not enough to make penetration comfortable or to make intercourse sustainable for more than a few minutes. The ass does not produce its own lubrication, so for anal play, lubrication is an absolute necessity. Even when your play does not include vaginal or anal penetration, the idea of a dry toy against the delicate, sensitive skin of the genitals just isn't as appealing as one with a dab of lube to smooth out any friction against the skin. So, when playing with toys such as vibrators, dildos, wands, anal toys, and penis pumps and sleeves, lube is an essential element to make the experience more pleasurable.

As a general rule, lube should feel good on and in your genitals. If you experience itching, burning, redness, or any kind of irritation, you likely have a sensitivity or allergy to one or more ingredients in the lube. Everyone's body responds differently to every lube. Don't be discouraged if your first lube adventure ends in a warm shower to rinse it off because it didn't feel good. You simply haven't found the right lube for you. You'll know when you do because it will feel warm, wet, and comfortable. Choosing the right lube is a very personal choice. Your best bet is to get sample sizes of several different brands and try them out. You may also end up with a few you like, or one for vaginal intercourse and another for anal play. There are three basic types of lube: oil-based, water-based, and silicone, and each one is discussed in this chapter. Within each category, there are different kinds, including flavored, warming, and lubes with or without certain ingredients. Read labels carefully; if you're not sure what's in a lube, ask the retailer or write to the manufacturer.

Why It's Best to Give Certain Anal Lubricants a Pass

Anal Eze is one of many lubes (often with very similar names) marketed as made especially for anal sex, to make it easier and more comfortable. These desensitizing lubes contain benzocaine (or a similar ingredient), a topical anesthetic—think Orajel for your butt. They numb your butt so you can't feel what's going on. When you use them, you're more likely to go farther or take something bigger into your ass than you're ready for. The result: a sore ass, possible tearing and damage to the delicate lining of the anal canal and rectum, and pain—all things that aren't exactly going to make you want to rush right out and try anal sex again. Whatever you slide into the ass will also get numb (not a good idea, either). Plus, if there is any pleasure to be had, you won't be able to feel it! Desensitizing lubes reinforce the myth that anal penetration *has* to be painful and that discomfort is inevitable. They are bad products with a bad message, and I never recommend them.

Irritated? Try Natural and Organic Lubes

Until recently, most water-based lubricants contained glycerin, a common ingredient that helps lube retain its consistency. However, glycerin is a kind of sugar, and yeast feeds on sugar, so many women find that these lubes can cause a vaginal yeast imbalance or a yeast infection. If you are especially prone to yeast infections, or you find that after having sex with a water-based lube, you begin to develop symptoms, you should consider a glycerin-free lube. Although glycerin is still on the ingredient list of many water-based lubes, luckily, manufacturers responded to women's needs for an alternative. There are a growing number of glycerin-free lubes on the market, including Frolic, Gun Oil H2O, HydraSmooth, Liquid Silk, Maximus, and Slippery Stuff.

In addition to concerns about glycerin, in recent years, there has been growing concern about the safety of parabens. Parabens are petroleum-based chemicals that discourage the growth of bacteria, and they are commonly used as preservatives in cosmetics, beauty products, and lubricants.

Some studies have linked parabens to weight gain, skin problems, and certain types of cancer. If you are concerned about parabens, read labels carefully (benzyl, butyl, ethyl, isobutyl, methyl, and propyl are all parabens). Several lubricant makers offer glycerin-free and paraben-free varieties, including Astroglide Glycerin/Paraben Free, ID Moments, Ride, Sliquid (all varieties), and Wet Naturals for Women.

Just as there has been a growing movement to buy food and beauty products with natural ingredients and without harmful chemicals, many consumers want their lube to be as natural as possible. If you're looking for lube with fewer chemical ingredients, try these water-based lubes:

- **O'My** contains ginseng, guarana, and gamiana, along with hemp seed extract, which moisturizes and discourages the growth of yeast, bacteria, and fungi.

- **Hathor Aphrodisia** is glycerin-free and contains natural botanical emollients.

- **Good Clean Love** is 95 percent organic and includes organic vegetable glycerin (which does not encourage yeast growth like synthetic glycerin), aloe vera, seaweed, herbs, and flowers.

- **Sliquid Organics** are glycerin-free and paraben-free lubes blended with certified organic botanicals, aloe vera, vitamin E, and green tea, and they come in earth-friendly packaging (the bottles are 100 percent recyclable).

- **Sensua Organics** contain organic aloe vera, organic grapefruit seed extract, wildcrafted and pesticide-free guar gum, and organic fruit flavors and fragrances (there is also an unflavored version).

- **Yes** is glycerin-free, paraben-free, and certified organic, and contains pure plant extracts.

- **Babeland Naturals** contain 95 percent organic ingredients, including vegetable glycerin and herbs.

Oil-Based Lubes: Good, but Not for Everything (or Everyone)

People often write to me and ask me whether it's safe to use common household products for lubrication during masturbation or partnered sex. Products such as lotion, baby oil, Vaseline, Abolene, massage oil, and olive oil are among the favorites. The biggest issue with all these items is that they contain some kind of oil or combination of oils. Oil is difficult, if not impossible, to clean up: It stains sheets and fabric, making it the least ideal for sex play. It also breaks down latex, which can cause microscopic holes or obvious tears in condoms; if you're practicing safer sex with latex condoms, gloves, or dental dams, oil-based lube makes them ineffective. It can degrade and ruin your favorite toys because it's not compatible with many sex toy materials. But the most important thing to know is that oil-based lubes aren't nice to vaginas! If any lube gets inside one, it's impossible to clean it up: You can't rinse or douche it out. It will linger in a vagina, providing an ideal environment for bacteria to grow. The result: a vaginal infection, an unhappy vagina, and no playtime for the vagina until the infection is treated.

You may spot oil-based lubricants in your favorite sex shop and wonder, if these are so bad for sex, why are they here? They aren't bad for all kinds of sex; oil-based lubes work best for male masturbation and hand jobs. In fact, some men say they prefer to masturbate with an oil-based lube because it doesn't get sticky and lasts a long time. Most oil-based lubes on the market contain mineral oil, coconut oil, almond oil, vegetable oil, or some combination. Many of them are formulated with ingredients so they won't stain fabrics (read the label carefully). Gun Oil is a popular brand, and the company makes several other oil-based lubes, including Jack Jelly and Stroke 29. Other brands include Boy Butter, Elbow Grease, Eros Power Cream, ID Cream, Men's Cream, Swiss Navy Cream, and Wet Oil Based Body Glide. Although they may be easier to clean up than household products, the rest of the rules apply: Oil-based lubes are not compatible with and should not be used with latex, many toys, and vaginas. You should reserve them for men's solo play. Or, if you are going to use them for a hand job during partnered sex, if you want to have intercourse or any kind of penetration afterward, make sure you wash the lube off his hands, your hands, and his penis, then switch to another kind of lube.

Water-Based Lubes: Safe, Clean, and Versatile

The majority of lubricants on the market are water-based. Water-based lubes are nonstaining, easy to clean up, and come in a variety of brands with different ingredients, consistencies, and tastes. They are compatible with all sex toy materials as well as safer sex barriers such as latex and nonlatex condoms. Popular brands include Astroglide, Durex, K-Y, ID Glide, Pink Water, Probe, Swiss Navy H2O, System JO H2O, and Wet.

Water-based lubes cover the spectrum in terms of consistency: They can be thin and liquidy, medium thickness, or super thick like hair gel. Thin, slippery lubes are meant to mimic vaginal fluids, and work well for vaginal penetration, while thicker lubes tend to stay wet longer and work better for anal penetration. The most common complaint about this kind of lube is that it tends to become sticky, stringy, or tacky as time goes by; it also dries up, because it gets absorbed into genital tissue. So, you need to relubricate—by adding saliva, water, or more lube—several times, which for some people breaks up the momentum of sex.

Keep in mind that if you plan on putting your mouth where your hands, toys, or a penis has been, you should select a lube you don't mind the taste of. Some water-based lubes, for example, have a bitter or chemical taste that really turns people off. If taste is a big issue for you, choose a flavored lube.

Spice It Up with Flavored Water-Based Lubes

Are you someone who doesn't stick to one sexual activity for a very long time? Do you like to switch things up frequently, moving from fingers, to oral, to toys, to a little more oral, add some more fingers, and . . . you get the idea. The last thing your lover wants to see is your head pop up from between her legs with an awful look on your face. If your mouth is frequently in the mix and you're using plenty of lube, you may want to consider a flavored lube because you're going to be tasting it often. Many of the major brands of lube have a flavored variety (or varieties), including Astroglide, ID, O'My, Sliquid, Swiss Navy, System JO, and Wet.

I have taste-tested most of the flavored lubes, and they aren't exactly yummy confections—many of them are chemical, artificial tastes akin to swallowing cold medicine. One of the biggest issues is that their taste isn't delicate, so you tend to either love it or hate it. For my money, Sliquid makes the most subtle, palatable flavored lubes, and their Blue Raspberry and Green Apple are my favorites (Green Apple is also their best-selling flavor, so it's not just me!).

Get the Best of Both Worlds with Hybrid Lubes

Liquid Silk and Sliquid Silk Hybrid Formula are water-silicone hybrid lubes: They combine the easy-to-clean, nonstaining properties of a glycerin-free water-based lube with the staying power of a silicone lube. Liquid Silk is safe to use with most silicone toys. Sliquid Silk Hybrid Formula is 12 percent silicone and doesn't contain parabens. Although the manufacturers play it safe and recommend you don't use them with silicone toys, some people say it's safe with the best-quality silicone (such as Vixen and Tantus).

Tips for a Quick Cleanup

When you use a lot of lube, sometimes it gets everywhere and you want a quick solution to clean it up, but you want something safe for those delicate parts of your body. You can use unscented alcohol-free baby wipes or wipes marked especially for sex, such as Pleasure Wipes and Afterglow Wipes.

Make It Hotter with Warming Lubes

One of the latest trends in the water-based lube marketplace is lube that creates a warming sensation on contact, and nearly all the major brands have produced one. The main ingredient differs: It might be acacia honey or a derivative (as in Astroglide Warming Liquid, Wet Warming Lubricant, and K-Y Warming Liquid), menthol (as in ID Sensation, Hot Elbow Grease, and the glycerin-free Sliquid Sizzle), or, the most natural of them all, cinnamon bark (in Emerita OH). When you apply these lubes to your genitals, they create a warming sensation that sends blood rushing to the area, which helps the arousal process. As with lube in general, whether you like it is totally a matter of personal preference. Some people find the sensation to be subtle and they love how it makes their private parts tingle. Some women find that it helps them get turned on faster. Others say the feeling is similar to sticking Bengay in your vagina or butt—it's way too intense and feels more annoying than pleasurable. Some people like these warming lubes for vaginal penetration but find the feeling too overwhelming for anal penetration.

Stay Slick with Silicone Lubes

Lubricants made with silicone are gaining in popularity and include such brands as Eros, Eros Gel, Astroglide X, Swiss Navy Silicone, System JO Original, Sliquid Silver, Gun Oil, Wet Platinum, K-Y Intrigue, and ID Velvet. Silicone lubes are nonstaining and often flavorless; they are more expensive than water-based ones, but you use a lot less of them because they don't dry up as easily. They tend to be super-concentrated and a little bit goes a long way. Many people prefer the slick texture of silicone and the fact that it doesn't get sticky or tacky, as some water-based lubes can. Silicone lubes work with condoms and other safer-sex barriers as well as some sex toy materials, including PVC, rubber, glass, hard plastic, acrylic, and metal. However, silicone lubes are NOT compatible with CyberSkin or silicone sex toys and will ruin them. So if you're a fan of these sex toy materials, you either need to cover your toys with condoms to protect them or use a different kind of lube. Silicone lube is perfect for sex in a shower or bath because it stays slick underwater, while water-based lubes don't.

Best Sellers: Top Lubes by Brand Name

Astroglide, astroglide.com

Eros, erosgel.com

Good Clean Love, goodcleanlove.com

ID, idlube.com

K-Y, k-y.com

Liquid Silk and Maximus, liquidsilk.com

Pink, empoweredproducts.com

Pjur, pjurusa.com

Slippery Stuff, slipperystufflube.com

Sliquid, sliquid.com

Swiss Navy, swissnavylube.com

System JO, systemjo.com

Wet, wetinternational.com

CHAPTER 22

TOY CARE, CLEANING, AND SAFETY

Practicing Safer Sex

Just because a sex toy is an inanimate object doesn't mean you cannot catch something from it! When we use sex toys, they may come into contact with many of your and your partner's bodily fluids, including semen, vaginal fluids, female ejaculate, rectal bacteria, and even fecal matter and blood. These fluids carry sexually transmitted infections (STIs), which can be passed on when one partner comes into contact with an infected partner's fluids. It's difficult—and, in the case of some STIs, very rare—for people to transmit an STI through sharing sex toys, because most STIs do not live very long outside the body, but it is possible. Thinking about all these fluids and infection may not sound sexy, but you need to think about safer sex practices when using sex toys.

Let's say you are in a monogamous relationship, have tested negative for all sexually transmitted infections—gonorrhea, chlamydia, syphilis, herpes, HPV, hepatitis, and HIV—and regularly have unprotected sex with your partner. You can share a nonporous toy with a partner after you clean and disinfect it. If it's an anal toy, you should still sanitize it. If you don't know your own or your partner's STI status, then you should practice safer sex to protect yourself, including playing with toys safely. If a toy is made of a porous material, then you should either not share it or put a new condom on it each time you use it. If a toy is made of a nonporous material, as long as you sterilize it, you can share it. Play safe!

Care and Cleaning

The key to maintaining your toys and having them last a long time is to care for them like you would any other important tools: Clean, care for, and store them properly. For rechargeable toys, always follow the charging instructions that come with them; usually, you must fully charge the toy when you get it home before you use it. Some vibrators, such as the Form 6, require a full 8 hours of charging time when you first get it, so make sure you plan ahead! I like to label the charger plug for each specific toy with a piece of tape, so that I don't get all my different chargers confused! Always store your battery-operated toys with the batteries removed, and make sure you change old batteries promptly. There's nothing worse than running out of juice just when you need it most! Vibrators tend to drain batteries quickly, so I recommend top-quality name-brand alkaline batteries; off-brand batteries that come free with toys are often lower quality and shouldn't be used. Follow instructions about putting batteries in a toy, because most toys require a specific configuration for them to work properly.

People have different opinions about and experiences with using regular batteries or the kind you can recharge. Some say that as long as you remove them after each use, rechargeable batteries work just as well as regular batteries. Others say that rechargeable batteries lose power faster or have less power to begin with, which is problematic for vibrators that need a lot, so these toys just don't run as well. Each time you charge them, rechargeable batteries can hold less power, which can cause them to die out quicker. Whichever you choose, the most important thing is, always have some more handy!

In discussing cleaning recommendations, I will make an important distinction: You can clean any toy (washing it for hygienic purposes) and you can sterilize some toys depending on what they're made of (so that they may be shared with someone). Educate yourself about what kind of toy you have and what it's made of. For example, a waterproof toy can be submerged in water, whereas a water-resistant toy won't be damaged by some water on it, but it cannot be submerged or soaked. When reading the following, note that no toys with electrical components should be soaked, boiled, or put in the dishwasher. These toys should be wiped down only. When storing your toys, keep them out of direct sunlight, away from heating sources, and in a place with some air circulation but not a lot of moisture.

Latex, PVC, vinyl, elastomer, TPR, and other soft materials: Because all of these materials are porous to some degree (with PVC and jelly rubber being the most porous), they can be cleaned but not sterilized. In other words, you can wash off lube, residue, and most bodily fluids, but some may linger in the nicks and minute crevices that are often present in these materials. Wash them with warm water and mild soap or use a sex toy cleaner. If you want to share one of these toys, you should cover it with a new condom for each partner.

CyberSkin: Not all thermal plastics are the same, so you should always follow the cleaning instructions that come with a toy. Many of the thermal plastics, (including the Real Feel Super Skin of the Fleshlight) require a two-step process. Right after you use the toy, you should rinse it with warm water only and allow it to air-dry thoroughly. Then, cover the entire thing with cornstarch—it must be cornstarch, not baby powder or talc—and dust off the excess. If you skip the cornstarch step, the toy becomes incredibly sticky, picking up dirt and lint instantly! Store it in a cool, dry place away from other toys, because other materials can often react with thermal plastic and melt it. Thermal plastics are porous, so you should not share these toys with other people; if you want to, cover them with a condom first.

Silicone: Unlike all other soft sex toy materials, medical-grade and platinum silicones are not porous, much easier to clean, and can be sterilized. You can clean them with hot water and antibacterial soap or a sex toy cleaner. You can sanitize them in a number of different ways. Let them soak for a few minutes in a diluted bleach solution of 10 parts water to 1 part bleach, then rinse them very well. You can put them in the top rack of the dishwasher without detergent or place them in boiling water for about 3 minutes. Allow them to air-dry, because drying them with any kind of towel often leads to lint clinging to the toys. Because these toys can be disinfected, they can be shared with other partners once they are thoroughly sanitized. Store them in a cool, dry place; they can be stored with other silicone toys, but shouldn't be in the same bag, box, or drawer with toys made of other soft materials. A bag or case lined with satin or another silky material is ideal for silicone, because it can easily pick up lint, dust, hair, and fuzz.

Hard plastics and acrylic: Hard plastics include resin, urethane, PVC (without softeners), and any other solid plastics; hard plastic toys run the gamut between those that are porous and those that aren't. All of them may be cleaned with warm water and a mild antibacterial soap or a sex toy cleaner. Unless the manufacturer states that the plastic is medical-grade and nonporous, assume that it cannot be sterilized. Caring properly for acrylic toys is very important if you want to maintain their crystal clear transparency and finish. They're nonporous and tough (nearly unbreakable), but they can be easy to scratch. To sterilize, soak them in a diluted bleach solution (10 parts water to 1 part bleach), then rinse them well. Don't boil them or run them through the dishwasher, and never wipe them down with alcohol because it will ruin the material by causing tiny cracks throughout it. Let acrylic air-dry thoroughly or use a very soft cloth—never use a paper towel or toilet paper, because they can scratch the surface. Store toys in something soft, such as a sock or a velvet or satin bag (which often comes with the toy). These toys are nonporous and can be shared after they're properly cleaned and disinfected.

Glass: Glass toys are also nonporous and can be used by different partners as long as you sterilize them. You can clean them with warm water and antibacterial soap or a sex toy cleaner and disinfect them by soaking them in a diluted bleach solution (10 parts water to 1 part bleach) or alcohol. Let them air-dry or wipe them down with a soft cloth. Although I recommend that you buy only Pyrex or borosilicate glass toys, there are toys on the market made of lesser grades of glass. If you know the toy is borosilicate glass, then you can put it in the top rack of the dishwasher without detergent on a gentle setting to sterilize it. Store each toy in its own separate soft bag to protect it, preferably a cushioned bag (which often

comes with the toy). Never put two glass toys in one bag, because they can bang together. Quality glass toys should be tough and resilient; however, if one ever develops a chip or nick, stop using it and throw it away immediately.

Aluminum, stainless steel, and other metals: Metal can be cleaned with warm water and antibacterial soap and sterilized with diluted bleach solution (10:1) or alcohol, or by washing in the top rack of the dishwasher without detergent. Metal toys must be dried completely to prevent rusting, especially those that are not one single piece but several joined together. Store metal toys away from light in their own soft bag or a sock to protect them from other toys, especially other hard materials such as glass.

Exotic materials: Throughout this book there have been mentions of unique, exotic, and luxury sex toy materials, including wood, ceramic, granite, gold, and platinum. For these and any other materials not listed here, always follow cleaning instructions from the manufacturer.

CHAPTER 23

BUILDING YOUR TOY BOX

Your Guide to Storage Solutions

It's important to keep your toys in a cool, dry place away from sunlight, dust, pet hair, and anything else that can prevent them from being clean. It's also a good idea to find somewhere safe to keep them out of sight from roommates, kids, pets, and anyone else who might be poking around. Children are endlessly curious about what's in their parents' bedroom, and if you're not ready to have the "What's a dildo?" discussion, then make sure you follow your own rule: Put your toys away. Dogs assume that all rubber toys are theirs, and when your shih tzu trots into the living room with a butt plug in her mouth during a party, you might be a little embarrassed (plus, now your butt plug has teeth marks in it). Some people have a special drawer in their nightstand for all their toys or a designated shelf in a cabinet or the closet. The Hide Your Vibe Pillow by Sportsheets has a hidden pocket designed to hold a favorite toy or two, and the Sugar Sak is a satin bag with a lining that inhibits the growth of mold, bacteria, and viruses.

If, like me, you have a sex toy collection that has grown too big for just one drawer, you have a few options. You can buy a large rectangular storage bin designed to go under the bed; this way, you can slide it out when you're ready to play and hide it away when you're done. Several companies specialize in storage solutions for your sex toys:

- **For Your Nymphomation (foryournymphomation.com):** This company has some of the most stylish, versatile, and well-designed cases and toy boxes, many designed for travel as well. From a small condom purse to a rolling toy trunk, the cases are made of faux leather with water-resistant nylon linings that are easy to clean. They have lots of ingenious little pockets and compartments that attach with Velcro and are interchangeable; plus, all the cases come with locks for added security. The zipper pulls glow in the dark, so they're easy to find when you're right in the middle of a hot encounter!

- **ToiBocks (toibocks.com):** Disguised as jewelry boxes, tissue box covers, and other common items that don't look out of place in a bedroom, these handcrafted wooden boxes are perfect for storing your favorite lube, safer sex supplies, DVDs, and a few toys.

- **Devine Toy Storage (devinetoys. com):** From the stylish Condom Cube to the Devine Satchel, Devine makes a line of storage products of faux crocodile skin and other fabrics.

Must-Have Items for Your Toy Box

- Lube
- Massage oil or bar
- Safer sex supplies
- Body wipes
- Sex toy cleaner
- Towel
- Batteries
- Erotic book or DVD
- Mouthwash or mints
- Extension cord

RESOURCE GUIDE

Books

The Adventurous Couple's Guide to Sex Toys by Violet Blue (San Francisco: Cleis Press, 2006).

The Adventurous Couple's Guide to Strap-On Sex by Violet Blue (San Francisco: Cleis Press, 2007).

Anal Pleasure and Health: A Guide for Men and Women by Jack Morin, PhD (San Francisco: Down There Press, 1998).

Becoming Orgasmic: A Sexual and Personal Growth Program for Women by Julia Heiman and Joseph LoPiccolo (New York: Fireside Books, 1987).

Dr. Sprinkle's Spectacular Sex: Make Over Your Love Life with One of the World's Great Sex Experts by Annie Sprinkle (New York: Tarcher/Penguin, 2005).

The Elusive Orgasm: A Woman's Guide to Why She Can't and How She Can Orgasm by Vivienne Cass (Cambridge, MA: Da Capo Press, 2007).

Em & Lo's Sex Toy: An A-Z Guide to Bedside Accessories by Em & Lo (San Francisco: Chronicle Books, 2006).

Female Ejaculation and the G-Spot by Deborah Sundahl (Alameda, CA: Hunter House, 2003).

Getting Off: A Woman's Guide to Masturbation by Jamye Waxman (Berkeley, CA: Seal Press, 2007).

The Good Vibrations Guide to Sex: The Most Complete Sex Manual Ever Written by Cathy Winks and Anne Semans (San Francisco: Cleis Press, 2002).

Guide to Getting It On (5th ed.) by Paul Joannides (Waldport, OR: Goofy Foot Press, 2006).

Healing Sex: A Mind-Body Approach to Healing Sexual Trauma by Staci Haines (San Francisco: Cleis Press, 2007).

I Love Female Orgasm by Dorion Solot and Marshall Miller (Cambridge, MA: Da Capo Press, 2007).

The Many Joys of Sex Toys: The Ultimate How-to Handbook for Couples and Singles by Anne Semans (New York: Broadway Books, 2004).

Never Have the Same Sex Twice: A Guide For Couples by Alison Tyler (San Francisco: Cleis Press, 2008).

Nina Hartley's Guide to Total Sex by Nina Hartley with I. S. Levine (New York: Avery, 2006).

Orgasms for Two: The Joy of Partnersex by Betty Dodson (New York: Harmony Books, 2002).

Sex for One: The Joy of Selfloving by Betty Dodson (New York: Three Rivers Press, 1996).

Sex Toys 101: A Playfully Uninhibited Guide by Rachel Venning and Claire Cavanah (New York: Fireside, 2003).

SM 101: A Realistic Introduction by Jay Wiseman (Oakland, CA: Greenery Press, 1998).

Videos

Toygasms! The Insider's Guide to Sex Toys and Techniques by Sadie Allison (San Francisco: Tickle Kitty Press, 2003).

The Ultimate Guide to Anal Sex for Men by Bill Brent (San Francisco: Cleis Press, 2002).

The Ultimate Guide to Anal Sex for Women (2nd ed.) by Tristan Taormino (San Francisco: Cleis Press, 2006).

The Ultimate Guide to Sex and Disability by Miriam Kaufman, Cory Silverberg, and Fran Odette (San Francisco: Cleis Press, 2007).

The Ultimate Guide to Strap-on Sex by Karlyn Lotney (San Francisco: Cleis Press, 2000).

Bend Over Boyfriend directed by Shar Rednour (Fatale Video, 1998).

Bend Over Boyfriend 2: More Rockin', Less Talkin' directed by Shar Rednour and Jackie Strano (S.I.R. Video/Fatale Media, 1999).

Better Sex Video Series Volume 3: Erotic Sex Play & Beyond (Sinclair Intimacy Institute, 2005).

Celebrating Orgasm: Women's Private Selfloving Sessions directed by Betty Dodson (Betty Dodson, 1996).

The Expert Guide to Anal Sex directed by Tristan Taormino (Vivid-Ed, 2007).

The Expert Guide to Anal Pleasure for Men directed by Tristan Taormino (Vivid-Ed, 2009).

Nina Hartley's Advanced Guide to Sex Toys directed by Nina Hartley (Adam & Eve, 2001).

Nina Hartley's Guide to Masturbation directed by Ernest Greene (Adam & Eve, 2004).

Nina Hartley's Guide to Strap-on Sex directed by Ernest Greene (Adam & Eve, 2006).

The Orgasm Doctor directed by Betty Dodson (Betty Dodson, 2008).

Personal Touch #1: Toying with Pleasure directed by Jamye Waxman (Adam & Eve, 2007).

Selfloving: Portrait of a Woman's Sexuality Seminar directed by Betty Dodson (Betty Dodson, 2005).

Toys for Better Sex (Sinclair Intimacy Institute, 2002).

Stores

The following are a selection of sex-positive retail sex toy stores. Many of them are women-owned and run, and all are women- and couples-friendly.

A Little More Interesting
alittlemoreinteresting.com
1501B 17th Avenue SW
Calgary, Alberta T2T 0E2
Canada
403-475-7775

Aphrodite's Toy Box
aphroditestoybox.com
3040 N. Decatur Road
Scottdale, GA 30079
404-292-9700

Art of Loving
artofloving.ca
1819 West Fifth Avenue
Vancouver, British Columbia V6J 1P5
Canada
604-742-9988

A Woman's Touch
a-womans-touch.com
888-621-8880
600 Williamson Street
Madison, WI 53703
608-250-1928

200 N. Jefferson Street
Milwaukee, WI 53202
414-221-0400

Babeland
babeland.com
800-658-9119
707 East Pike Street
Seattle, WA 98122
206-328-2914

94 Rivington Street
New York, NY 10002
212-375-1701

43 Mercer Street
New York, NY 10013
212-966-2120

462 Bergen Street
Brooklyn, NY 11217
718-638-3820

Coco de Mer
Coco-de-mer.com
23 Monmouth Street
Covent Garden
London WC2H 9DD
+44 (0)20 7836 8882

108 Draycott Avenue
South Kensington
London SW3 3AE
+44 (0)20 7584 7615

8618 Melrose Avenue
Los Angeles, CA 90069
310-652-0311

Come As You Are
comeasyouare.com
701 Queen Street West
Toronto, Ontario M6J 1E6
Canada
877-858-3160

Early to Bed
early2bed.com
5232 N. Sheridan
Chicago, IL 60640
773-271-1219

Eros Boutique
erosboutique.com
581A Tremont Street
Boston, MA 02118
866-425-0345

Fascinations
fascinations.net
Stores throughout Arizona, Colorado, and Oregon
See website for locations

Forbidden Fruit
forbiddenfruit.com
512 Neches
Austin, TX 78701
800-315-2029

Good for Her
goodforher.com
175 Harbord Street
Toronto, Ontario M5S 1H3
Canada
416-588-0900

Good Vibrations
goodvibes.com
800-289-8423
603 Valencia Street
San Francisco, CA 94110
415-522-5460

1620 Polk Street
San Francisco, CA 94109
415-345-0400

2504 San Pablo Avenue
Berkeley, CA 94702
510-841-8987

308-A Harvard Street
Brookline, MA 02446
617-264-4400

Hysteria
hysteriashop.com
114 S. Broadway
Denver, CO 80209
303-733-3373

It's My Pleasure
4258 SE Hawthorne Boulevard
Portland, OR 97215
503-236-0505

JT's Stockroom
stockroom.com
2807 W. Sunset Boulevard
Los Angeles, CA 90026
800-755-8697

Miko
mikoexoticwear.com
268 Wickenden Street
Providence, RI 02903
401-421-9787

Nomia Boutique
nomiaboutique.com
24 Exchange Street, Suite 215
Portland, ME 04101
207-773-4774

Oh My: A Sensuality Shop
ohmysensuality.com
2c Conz Street
Northampton, MA 01060
413-584-9669

Passional Toys
passional.net
620 S. 5th Street
Philadelphia, PA 19147
215-829-4986

The Pleasure Chest
pleasurechest.com
156 Seventh Avenue South
New York, NY 10014
212-242-2158

3436 North Lincoln Avenue
Chicago, IL 60657
773-525-7151

7733 Santa Monica Boulevard
West Hollywood, CA 90046
323-650-1022

The Rubber Rose
therubberrose.com
3812 Ray Street
San Diego, CA 92104
619-296-7673

Self Serve Toys
selfservetoys.com
3904B Central Avenue SE
Albuquerque, NM 87108
505-265-5815

Smitten Kitten
smittenkittenonline.com
3010 Lyndale Avenue South
Minneapolis, MN 55408
888-751-0523

Spartacus
spartacusstore.com
300 SW 12th Avenue
Portland, OR 97205
503-224-2604

Stormy Leather
stormyleather.com
1158 Howard Street
San Francisco, CA 94103
800-486-9650

Sugar
sugartheshop.com
927 W. 36th Street
Baltimore, MD 21211
410-467-2632

The Tool Shed
toolshedtoys.com
2427 N. Murray Avenue
Milwaukee, WI 53211
414-906-5304

Tulip Toy Gallery
mytulip.com
1480 W. Berwyn Avenue
Chicago, IL 60640
877-70-TULIP

Venus Envy
venusenvy.ca
1598 Barrington Street
Halifax, Nova Scotia B3J 1Z6
Canada
902-422-0004

320 Lisgar Street
Ottawa, Ontario K2P 0E2
Canada
613-789-4646

Wink
winkkc.com
1415 W. 39th Street
Kansas City, MO 64111
816-931-WINK

Womyns' Ware
womynsware.com
896 Commercial Drive
Vancouver, British Columbia V5L 3Y5
Canada
604-254-2543

Sex Toy Retail Websites

AdamEve.com

AllGlassSexToys.com

Blowfish.com

EdenFantasies.com

ExtremeRestraints.com

GlassFantasy.com

LiberatorShapes.com

Libida.com

MyPleasure.com

SexSwingStore.com

Sportsheets.com

Vibrator.com

Xandria.com

Sex Toy Home Party Companies

Athena's Home Novelties
(athenashn.com)

Bedroom Magic
(bedroommagic.com)

Booty Parlor Parties
(bootyparlorparties.com)

Essence of Romance
(essenceofromance.com)

For Your Pleasure
(foryourpleasure.com)

Just A Little Naughty
(justalittlenaughty.com)

Intimate Expressions
(intimate-expressions.com)

Passion Parties
(passionparties.com)

Pure Romance
(pureromance.com)

Slumber Parties
(slumberparties.com)

Top Sex Toy Brands

Aneros: prostate toys
Aneros.com

Aslan Leather: strap-on harnesses, bondage toys
AslanLeather.com

Big Teaze Toys: disguised, hands-free, unique vibrators
BigTeazeToys.com

California Exotic Novelties: large mainstream adult novelty company
CalExotics.com

Doc Johnson: large mainstream adult novelty company
DocJohnson.com

Eroscillator: Eroscillator vibrators
Eroscillator.com

Fleshlight: Fleshlight penis sleeves
Fleshlight.com

For Your Nymphomation: sex toy storage solutions
ForYourNymphomation.com

Fun Factory: silicone vibrators, dildos, butt toys
FunFactory.de

Jimmyjane: luxury sex toys and accessories
Jimmyjane.com

Jollies: silicone dildos, butt plugs, vibrating dildos, cock rings
JolliesPleasureToys.com

Kegelcisor: vaginal barbells
Kegelcisor.com

Lelo: luxury vibrators, cock rings, prostate toys
Lelo.com

Natural Contours: ergonomic, compact, and wand vibrators
Natural-Contours.com

Nectar Products: Crystal Wand
LoveNectar.com

Nexus: prostate and G-spot toys
NexusProstateMassagers.com

Njoy: stainless steel dildos, wands, and plugs
NjoyToys.com

Nob Essence: wooden dildos and wands
NobEssence.com

OhMiBod: MP3- and cell phone-compatible vibrators
OhMiBod.com

One Up Innovations: Liberator Shapes
LiberatorShapes.com

Pipedream: large mainstream adult novelty company
PipedreamProducts.com

Phallix: glass toys
PhallixGlass.com

PyreXions: glass toys
Pyrexions.com

Rocks Off: dual-action G-spot and P-spot vibrators
rocks-off.uk.com

Sportsheets: bondage toys, harnesses, accessories
Sportsheets.com

Stormy Leather: harnesses, bondage toys, leatherwear
StormyLeather.com

Tantus: silicone and metal toys
TantusSilicone.com

Topco: large mainstream adult novelty company
TopcoSales.us

Vibratex: dual-action and compact vibrators
Vibratex.com

Vixen Creations: silicone dildos, butt plugs, toys
VixenCreations.com

We-Vibe: We-Vibe wearable vibrator
We-Vibe.com

Sex Ed Websites

Dodsonandross.com
This is the online home of author, sexologist, and masturbation coach Betty Dodson and sex-positive activist Carlin Ross.

Nina.com
Adult film star and sex educator Nina Hartley's official website contains message boards where you can ask questions about anal sex and information about her sex ed video series.

Puckerup.com
Tristan Taormino's sex advice website contains an archive of hundreds of questions and answers about anal sex, information about her books and videos, and sex advice message boards.

Sexuality.org
Founded by the Society for Human Sexuality, this website contains an abundance of articles, advice, and resources for all things sexual.

Sfsi.org
Got a question you're too embarrassed to ask anyone else? San Francisco Sex Information to the rescue! This nonprofit organization's website offers free, confidential, accurate, nonjudgmental information about sex.

Tinynibbles.com
Sex educator and author Violet Blue's website contains smart, sexy advice on all things sexual, including sex toys.

Vivid-Ed.com
The educational imprint of Vivid Entertainment Group, Vivid-Ed produces sex ed videos for a new generation.

ACKNOWLEDGMENTS

I want to thank Jill Alexander, Rosalind Wanke, John Gettings, Jennifer Grady, Susan Hershberg, Karen Levy, Christina Antoniades, Will Kiester, and everyone at Quiver Books for their hard work on this book. Thanks to all the fantastic models and to Luciana Pampalone for her gorgeous and inspired photography. Thanks to Cory Silverberg from Come As You Are in Toronto for his contribution to the book and Sarah Sloane and Colten Tognazzini for all their assistance.

Several amazing companies sent us the majority of the toys and accessories which appear in the book, and I want to thank them: Tony Levine and Pamela McKee at Big Teaze Toys (bigteazetoys.com) for the Onye and Tuyo; Greg DeLong of NJoy (njoytoys.com) for the gorgeous metal toys; Vixen Creations (vixencreations.com) for the silicone dildos and plugs; Carrie Gray at Aslan Leather (aslanleather.com) for the strap-on harnesses; Jordan at Bonkum (bonkum.com) for the amazing Bonk'er; Inge at Advanced Response Corporation for the Eroscillator (eroscillator.com); Don Cohen at OneUp Innovations for the Liberator Shapes (liberatorshapes.com); Deanna Moen at Jimmyjane (Jimmyjane.com) for the Form 6 and the Iconic Ring; Alisa Richmond at Vibratex (vibratex.com) for the vibrators; John Richardson at Aneros (aneros.com) for the prostate toys; Amy Pomering at Outlaw Leather (outlawseattle.com) for the strap-on harness; Emily at Sportsheets (sportsheets.com); Betty Dodson (bettydodson.com) for Betty's Barbell; Hilda Brownlee from Standard Innovation Corporation for the We-Vibe (we-vibe.com); Pamela from Babeland for the SaSi (babeland.com); Alicia from NobEssence (nobessence.com) for the wooden toys; Coyote Days at Good Vibrations for the vibrators and bath goodies (goodvibes.com); Dawn at ToiBocks (toibocks.com) for the wooden storage box; Mario from JT's Stockroom (stockroom.com); and the folks at OhMiBod (ohmibod.com).

ABOUT THE AUTHOR

Tristan Taormino is an award-winning author, columnist, editor, sex educator, and adult film director. She is the author of five books: *The Anal Sex Position Guide*, *Opening Up: Creating and Sustaining Open Relationships*, *True Lust: Adventures in Sex, Porn and Perversion*, *Down and Dirty Sex Secrets*, and *The Ultimate Guide to Anal Sex for Women*. She wrote the popular *Village Voice* syndicated sex column "Pucker Up," for more than nine years, and she is a columnist for *Hustler's Taboo*. She is the creator and original series editor of *Best Lesbian Erotica*, which has won three Lambda Literary Awards. She runs her own adult film production company, Smart Ass Productions, and has directed more than a dozen adult films. She is currently an exclusive director for Vivid Entertainment. For Vivid, she directs a reality series called *Chemistry* and the vignette series *Rough Sex*, and helms its sex education imprint, Vivid-Ed, for which she has written, produced, and directed several titles, including *The Expert Guide to Anal Sex*, *The Expert Guide to Oral Sex 1: Cunnilingus*, *The Expert Guide to Oral Sex 2: Fellatio*, and *The Expert Guide to the G-Spot*. Tristan has been featured in more than two hundred publications; has appeared on CNN, HBO's *Real Sex*, *The Howard Stern Show*, *Loveline*, *Ricki Lake*, MTV, Fox News, The Discovery Channel; and has been on more than six dozen radio shows. She lectures on sexuality, gender, feminism, and pornography at top colleges and universities, including Brown, Cornell, Columbia, Sarah Lawrence, Yale, Vassar, Smith, Wesleyan, New York University, University of California/Santa Barbara, and University of Wisconsin/Milwaukee. She teaches sex and relationship workshops around the world and runs two websites, Puckerup.com and Openingup.net. She lives in upstate New York with her partner and their three dogs.